THE CONSUMER'S GUIDE
TO DENTAL IMPLANTS

Quiz:
What is Most
Important to You
in Selecting
an Implant
Dentist?

3 KEYS EVERY ADULT NEEDS
TO KNOW ABOUT A
SMILE TRANSFORMATION

BY DR. TYLER WILLIAMS, D.D.S.

outskirts
press

This book is dedicated to my many wonderful patients who have experienced the benefits of the dental implant revolution. I thank my beautiful wife, Megan, and my three wonderful children for their support throughout my career. It's been an interesting ride with ups and downs, but I am so glad we have done this together. I wouldn't be where I am without you all.

I thank God for the ability to help me learn and to understand the growing field of dentistry and how it can transform the lives of my patients.

Table of Contents

Introduction

Are you unhappy with your smile? Would you like to touch-up or improve the appearance, function, or color of your teeth? Or, are you looking to radically change or makeover your entire smile? If any of the above is what you are looking for, then this book is just what the doctor ordered. Today, the dental implant revolution is changing lives and improving patients' health everywhere you go. As medical costs continue to rise, more and more research is being done on the health benefits of dental implants, as well as the connection of the mouth to the entire body. I've had countless examples of experiences in my own practice of patients who have improved the health of their mouth and seen their general and specific health problems improve.

As an example, I'll share a story about my patient "Julie." Julie is fictional, but her example is very realistic. Julie had a few teeth removed in her late 20s because it seemed too complex or expensive to save them at the time. They were back teeth and she could still eat OK, and nobody noticed them. Several decades later, she was forced with the decision to save or remove additional teeth, as her bite had shifted and she had developed a few problems in some other back teeth.

What should she do?

She now has the choice to save her remaining teeth, remove them, or replace the missing ones. Any of these three choices could be right for Julie. Now, consider if she has more teeth removed and does nothing else. Back teeth continue to shift and front teeth begin to shorten and get rough edges, because they are getting too much force on them. Julie eats a softer and more refined diet, because she can't chew coarse vegetables or natural foods very well. Now she develops diabetes and high blood pressure which further complicates the issues in her gums.

If this is you, you likely can reverse or restore many of these issues. Don't feel bad; there are tens of thousands of people out there just like you. We have helped many of them.

If you haven't gone down this path, this book will help you avoid most of, if not all of, these problems going forward.

As we know, chronic diseases such as cancer, diabetes, and heart disease are on the rise. These diseases have a close and important link with the health of our mouth and gums. You may be asking yourself questions. Should you save your teeth or have them replaced? Straighten or implants? Does teeth whitening really work? Whether you are looking for a quick boost in the way you feel about your smile, or if you're looking to capture the smile you've dreamed about for years, I've written this book to help you understand your options and to be able to decide what is right for you and how to approach it. The transformation possibilities are up to you.

This book is composed of many mini-chapters. We have put it together this way for you to be able to quickly navigate the most relevant and helpful information to you. When you need to reference this book again, the information will be easy to locate. This way you can start taking action to discover the implant options that are best for you, and start improving your dental health starting today.

Section 1:
A Healthier Foundation

ONE

Build Your Foundation on Solid Rock

Do you remember the old song about the wise man who built his house upon the rock? As a child, this song greatly impacted the way I thought about and understood the importance of a solid foundation. I used to be terrified of the wind and rain because I watched *The Wizard of Oz* as a child and was worried my house was going to blow away, so when I heard this song, it made me think about how the storms of life can come down and beat upon us. That's the key point. Whether your house is built upon rock or sand will not prevent the storms from coming. Your mouth is no different. You experience oral health challenges every single day, from foods, beverages, mouth breathing, preservatives, medications (including supplements), and our home health routine paired with our professional dental visits.

If you have good teeth, you should not take them all out and replace them with dental implants. I repeat, if you have good teeth, do not remove them and replace them with dental implants. It's not a free ticket. Just like a high-end Mercedes Benz or Cadillac, dental implants require maintenance and care, just as regular teeth do. A high-performance vehicle may even require additional maintenance. However, if you have missing teeth or teeth in very poor health, then replacing them with dental implants or newer restorative options may be the way to go for you.

In this book, I'll discuss the three keys to getting the smile of your dreams so you can decide with the checklist and self-assessments provided, as well as some basic knowledge about the principles of your mouth, to help you figure out the direction you should go and to decide how to care for it in the long-term. I call these three options **refresh, restore and replace**.

Medical expenses are skyrocketing. We all know that medical expenses go up year after year. Our current healthcare crisis is a concern for millions of Americans. The popular question, "Will my insurance cover that?" is asked every single day at doctors' offices and hospitals everywhere. Many employers are now opting for high-deductible plans. Although this may be different than what you were used to in the past, I think it's a great move. Why? Because this places the decision of care in the hands of the patients and consumers, like you, who can make the best decisions regarding their own health.

Several years ago, I also opted for an independent high-deductible plan, which has helped me and my family better understand why and what we are receiving in terms of our own healthcare. But, how does our mouth tie into this? Is going to the dentist different than going to your family doctor or specialist? Why is dentistry not always part of mainstream healthcare? The distinction may be in regards to our training, because dentists are trained in independent schools and do not go through the same medical programs that physicians and surgeons go through. That could be part of it. But, I think the bigger reason for this has to do with third-party benefits and insurance coverage.

Our world's become very driven and dictated by what our "insurance will cover." Since my deductible is nearly $8,000, I completely understand and appreciate this, because costs are typically of some concern. But, I also find that we often make decisions based too much on what our insurance will cover and not on what is right for us. For example, tests, scans, and laboratory procedures that should be done are different than those that could be done. It's up to us to be informed and to make the right decision regarding our health.

Nearly 50% of Americans are without dental insurance, which means that half of my own patients have their own questions, because they may think they can't get a certain procedure done or see me for preventative care because they don't have coverage. This thought is completely misleading because we know that preventative care saves millions of dollars in America every year. In fact, hundreds of millions of work and school hours are lost annually in the U.S. alone due to dental illness or toothaches. Studies have also shown that when our mouth is healthy, our medical expenses are reduced by 21% or more overall. That's a pretty big number to me. That means I could shave off almost a quarter of my family's medical expenses when I ensure that our mouths stay healthy. That's my responsibility and obligation to my family and to the people of my community, just like you.

TWO

Periodontal Health, the Core of Your Smile

Today, nearly 50% of adults have periodontal disease, which includes gingivitis. That number jumps up to nearly 75% in seniors. Periodontal disease is the number one reason for tooth loss, but with early intervention and care, we can save most or all of your teeth. On my mom's side of the family, we have genetic history of periodontal disease. Both my mom's parents wore dentures and lost most of their teeth at an early age. This was back when teeth were usually pulled instead of being replaced if there was any doubt the tooth would live to bite another day. Today, however, we have different methods of periodontal therapy that are more comfortable, more affordable, and simpler to do than ever. We also have many things you can do at home to keep your smile happy that only require a few minutes each day.

Just like a good exercise routine keeps our body healthy, a good home routine will get our smile into shape and help us feel better than ever. Brushing is no longer enough. Today, tooth decay, or cavities as they are often called, is the number two chronic disease in the country, just behind the common cold. Although over 95% of us will experience tooth decay during our lifetime, it is a preventable disease. Over 2.1 billion dollars are spent each year on dental emergencies, according to the Centers for Disease Control. I despise when a tooth needs a root canal that could've been prevented, which is most of the time. Often, this is still the best choice, and saving the tooth is better than removing it.

However, when a tooth is severely cracked, broken, or decayed, more often than not nowadays, we will remove the tooth and replace it with an implant, and my patients, who are just like you, feel and chew great. In fact, dental implants feel and chew just like real teeth, and many people forget which tooth was the implant, because they look and feel so natural and real.

In our busy, on-the-go world, many of us only brush once a day, but even those who brush two times a day experience tooth decay. Dry mouth from medications, high starchy or sugar diets, and even energy and diet drinks are sabotaging the health of our mouths. As we live longer, it's important that we take special care of our teeth using soft brushes and the right kind of toothpaste to get our mouth healthy.

Sixty-six percent is not a great score. When we brush alone, we miss 1/3 of our tooth surface. Those tight and sometimes hard-to-reach areas between our teeth where food and bacteria love to hide are only cleaned well with flossing. Lately, there's been some controversy whether flossing is effective or not, but I can tell you from firsthand experience with my own patients, as well as research projects I did in dental school, and studies I have been involved in after, that dental floss works. Whether you use the bows with picks on them, or the regular, old-fashioned string floss, which is my preference, flossing once a day may be the most cost-effective thing you can do to save your teeth and to protect your pocketbook.

THREE

During Pregnancy

If you are female and have experienced the miracle of child-birth, you may have noticed bleeding gums during pregnancy. We call this pregnancy gingivitis. Due to increased blood flow throughout your body, your gums can become swollen and sensitive, bleed when flossing or brushing, and even cause bad breath.

If your gingivitis goes untreated, it can develop into periodontal disease, or gum disease as it's commonly known. Gum disease has been shown to decrease fertility in couples who are struggling to get pregnant, as well as increase the risk for heart disease and strokes.

Gum disease can lead to gestational diabetes as well as other conditions you won't want to add to all the other changes you experience during pregnancy. So, don't stop brushing or flossing while you're pregnant, and you are definitely safe and even encouraged to seek preventative dental care during pregnancy.

Every six months at a minimum, and every three or four months for a preventative visit if you are high risk or have gum disease. Even modern digital dental X-rays are safe if they are used to screen or rule out tooth decay and/or gum disease. Not only will it make you more comfortable and help you maintain your smile, but it can make the difference in keeping your baby safe before and during childbirth.

In their book *YOU: Having a Baby*, Dr. Mehmet Oz ("Dr. Oz") and Dr. Michael Roizen, MD, stress that if you have gum disease while pregnant, you are "seven times more likely to have babies born too early and born too small." That's not a typo: seven times more likely.

They further elaborate that the bacteria trapped between your teeth can get into your bloodstream, and it's magnified by estrogen, which can cause narrowing and inflammation of your arteries.

FOUR

The Secret Combination of Xylitol and Fluoride

To be clear, xylitol and fluoride are very different, but they're also very effective when used together. Fluoride is a naturally-occurring mineral in the earth. Fluoride in the water has been very controversial, but I won't go into detail on that here. The type of fluoride I'm talking about is a fluoride varnish, which can be applied to your teeth, or the topical fluoride found in toothpaste. These are very safe, because they're applied directly to your teeth, and you spit the extra away or brush it off.

Fluoride in the water only impacts developing children till about the age 12. Beyond that, fluoride in the water doesn't really help our teeth much. But, a fluoride varnish applied to your teeth in a professional dental office can provide three to six months of benefits, plus daily use of an effective fluoride toothpaste can help put calcium and minerals back into your teeth.

I strive for three calcium and fluoride exposures per day in my mouth. My home routine goes something like this: When I wake up, I rinse my mouth with a calcium mouthwash. After breakfast, I brush my teeth, then I spit out the extra toothpaste, and I avoid eating, drinking, or rinsing for 20 minutes. This way, it leaves behind the fluoride minerals on my teeth to recharge my enamel and decrease sensitivity. Then, I brush a second time before bed, and I do the same, avoiding eating, drinking, or rinsing for 20 minutes afterward. This has dramatically cut down on the sensitivity of my teeth, and it has also helped keep me cavity-free for over eight years and counting.

Xylitol is derived from natural sugar that comes from plants and trees. The great thing about xylitol is it contains half the calories of real sugar, and it's safe for children and adults, as well as people with certain medical conditions, such as diabetes. Just keep it away from your pets, especially dogs. Their stomachs can't process it. Xylitol tastes just like real sugar, only it is very gentle to our teeth and helps turn off bacteria that can cause tooth decay, as well as bacteria that can cause nose and sinus issues. Replacing your table sugar with small amounts of xylitol just might be the key to a healthier smile, as well as cutting down on calories.

FIVE

Water, the Free and Easy Way to Ensure Your Smile Lasts a Lifetime

A few years ago, a study came out that found that in the US, over 51% of our calories are consumed in liquid form. That's alarming. That means that we're getting over half our calories from drinking soft drinks, shakes, smoothies, or other liquid foods. The problem with this is most of these are very refined and processed, which means they stick to our teeth, and because we're not chewing them, they can stay there longer than they should. Drinking water is real insurance. Today, diet drinks are becoming more popular, including sugar-free energy drinks. These contain synthetic sugars that have many preservatives in them and can be very acidic. They're not good for our body and haven't shown to be beneficial to our teeth either. I can't tell you how many soda drinkers I see in a week, including diet soda drinkers, who have recurring and avoidable problems with their teeth.

Don't get me wrong, I love soda and my treats. I'm not going to say I never have them, but I limit them to small quantities and infrequently. Being a daily drinker of these harsh drinks can destroy a smile in a hurry and cost you thousands of dollars in root canals or in restoring teeth from problems that can be prevented and avoided altogether.

SIX

What's Your Frequency?

How often do you see the dentist for professional checkups? Think about this for a minute. Whether it's your car, your favorite hobby, or your exercise routine, think about how often you maintain and condition for these activities. My goal is to get the entire state to a dentist each year, but that alone isn't enough. Right now, too many people haven't been to the dentist for several years and problems are stockpiling. However, to get the best oral health possible, you should come in for professional cleanings two to four times per year.

Personally, I switched to three preventative care cleanings per year a year or so ago. I don't have a history of gum disease, but I've had braces, wisdom teeth removed, a crown, several chipped teeth, and even a few gum grafts for some of my sensitive receded gums. I decided to switch from seeing my hygienist twice a year to three times a year. (Just recently I increased my personal in-office maintenance to four times per year instead of three.) I realize that to maintain the teeth I've worked hard for, and to keep them bright and clean, that's what I need to do to be healthier. In fact, writing this chapter reminded me to schedule my complete checkup.

SEVEN

Why the Toothpaste Aisle at Your Local Pharmacy may be Missing Something

I'm often asked, "Which toothpaste or mouth rinse is the best? Should I use Brand X or Brand Y?" I've tried just about every rinse and toothpaste I could get my hands on, and I've also recommended different types over the years. If you really want to make a change, or get your mouth healthy, I suggest forgetting everything you find in the toothpaste aisle at the store. There are just too many preservatives, chemicals, and ingredients that are not beneficial to your mouth, and sometimes, there are even detrimental ingredients they don't tell you about on the label. The point of toothpaste and rinse is to gently clean away the plaque and bacteria that build up on our teeth, and to apply minerals to them. You don't need harsh chemicals to kill bacteria every time we brush or floss. This would be like using antibiotics to avoid a cold. It's overkill, and the risks can far outweigh the benefits.

Not all these products are bad, but it can be too hard to decide which one is right for you. If you really want to get a product to change your smile, I suggest finding things with simpler ingredients that contain a combination of xylitol and fluoride, and have neutral PH levels. Two brands I recommend are CariFree by Oral Biotech, which offers a prescription-strength toothpaste that can only be purchased through limited dental professionals, and Spry products by Xlear, which contain natural ingredients and fluoride that are gentle on our smiles and don't have the unnecessary ingredients and acidic preservatives that many long shelf-life products do.

By using these principles, as well as some basic common sense, and by managing your diet correctly, you should be able to maintain and strengthen the foundation of your smile. Dental implants are incredible, but as I often mention to my patients, the implants God gave you are often the best ones you can have. Plus, with newer technologies, there are hybrid or combination ways to incorporate dental implants while saving some or all of your remaining teeth that I'll go into later in detail in this book. For more checklists, reports, and information, visit the website contained in this book to get your bonus book extras.

EIGHT

"Gnashing of Teeth?" Stop the Daily Grind

Bruxism, or teeth grinding and clenching, is one of the most destructive forces on your teeth. Studies show it wears your teeth away ten or more times faster than regular eating. That means just one night of teeth grinding is equivalent to the amount of wear for eating during 1-2 weeks, depending on your severity!

This problem is as old as the Bible, when "gnashing of teeth" was used as an illustrative term to describe terrible sounds and destructive forces. It is the same today, a terrible sound, and for many, it's the beginning of the end for teeth.

"Bruxism" generally happens when you are asleep and/or stressed, so we can't usually stop it cold turkey. The good news is that you can minimize or eliminate the damage by changing lifestyle habits, by having a better sleep routine, by eating healthier and by protecting your teeth. The most effective option we have for this is an acrylic or resin custom-fitted mouthguard that we design right in the office pared with Botox treatments..

Think of wearing out the cartilage or socket on your knee or hip. Once that happens, it's either surgery or full replacement. Teeth work the same, only most people do not realize the damage because your enamel is so much harder than bone, and it doesn't have the nerves or sensation that other parts of your body do to send out a smoke signal when you are wearing it away, until it gets really bad!

I shared a story in my previous book, *Reason to Smile: 11 Keys to Your Best Oral Health Ever*, where one night while sleeping, I was startled by my lovely wife Megan grinding her teeth. This was just after we were married and a shock to both of us. I was surprised and concerned at the terrible noise and, like most people, she didn't understand the complexity at the time, but we took action immediately and her mouth has been much healthier ever since.

Take action by protecting your teeth today. It won't get better on its own, but get a customized guard made and/or Botox treatments from a qualified dentist, and work on ways to improve your lifestyle to reduce stress and to stay fit. You should also have any medical conditions such as heartburn and/or sleep apnea treated with the help of your physician.

NINE

TMJ...What Does it Mean?

TMJ is actually a misnomer, because we all have "TMJ." The tempromandibular joint is a rotating socket that connects both sides of your lower jaw to your skull. When people refer to TMJ, they usually mean TMJ disorder, or TMD (tempromandibular disorder), which can be very uncomfortable and problematic.

TMJ disorders are typically more common in women, people with a history of trauma or accidents on their jaw, sleep apnea or teeth grinding patients, people with worn, flat or missing teeth, and people with jaw development that is asymmetrical. If you injure your shoulder or knee joint, you can isolate it from the other side of your body. But your "TMJ" is the most complex and amazing joint in your body, because unlike most other joints, you can't move or open one jaw joint without opening the other.

We usually treat TMJ disorder with an appliance and Botox, home exercises, and therapy. Sometimes, we also involve a physical therapy, and Botox. Sometimes, we also involve a physical therapist or a chiropractor who is experienced with TMJ for in-office therapy. Our TMD appliances (which are different than appliances for teeth grinding alone) can really help the jaws and muscles relax into a more comfortable position that will help you relax and feel better.

TEN

Don't Lose Sleep Over it; Dental Health Meets Medical Health

Sleep apnea and snoring are the bridge between dental disease and medical conditions, and for many of my patients, getting sleep apnea treated makes all the difference in quality of life, and it cuts down dramatically on medical and dental expenses.

Bruxism and other medical conditions, such as diabetes, heartburn, TMD, heart disease, and even cancer, are tied in closely with our sleep health.

I have a family member who actually broke several of his implants over the years because he suffered with severe sleep issues, including sleep apnea. By treating it like any other chronic disease with follow-up therapy and daily appliance wear, we created a plan to manage his issues and to save his implants and smile.

ELEVEN

How Well are You Caring for Your Teeth?

Take this self-assessment to find out how well you are currently caring for your teeth.

Question 1: How often do you brush each day?

A) Zero times per day. B) One time per day. C) Two or more times per day.

Question 2: How long do you brush each time?

A) 30 seconds or less. B) One minute. C) Two minutes or less.

Question 3: How often do you floss?

A) Once per month or less. B) Once per week. C) Once per day or less.

Question 4: Do you smoke?

A) Yes. B) Sometimes. C) No.

Question 5: How often do you see the dentist?

A) Once every five years or more. B) Once per year.
C) Once every six months or more frequently.

Question 6: Do you have bleeding when you brush or floss?

A) Often. B) Sometimes. C) Never.

Question 7: Do you drink water between and with meals?

A) Rarely. B) Two to three times per week. C) Daily.

Question 8: Do you clench or grind your teeth at night?

A) Quiet often: You have sleep apnea, wake with headaches, wake with dry mouth, or your significant other says you grind and/or snore while sleeping. B) Yes, a few times per week. C) Never.

Score your results.

Each question marked A receives zero points.

Each question marked B receives one-half point.

Each question marked C receives one point.

Add up the totals.

0-3 total points: Let's work on your home routine. All health is connected to the health of many other systems in our bodies. Don't beat yourself up; now is the time for change. You can do it!

4-6 points: You're making progress. Keep working on that and you'll be an oral health pro in no time. For now add one or two goals for improvement.

7-8 points: Congrats, you're doing awesome. Keep up the great work.

Are you at risk for tooth decay?
Take this self-assessment to find out now.

How safe is your diet?

Research has found that eating coarse foods such as leafy greens and vegetables not only is great for your body but it provides vitamins to your mouth and gums and also helps naturally clean your teeth. There are vital nutrients in vegetables and dark fruits that help our bodies digest food, get the nutrition we need and help our mouths maintain a healthy pH (safe acidity level). Eat a diet low in processed foods and sugar, and high in the right types of natural foods, including proper proteins and healthy fats. It is also important to drink water instead of diet soda or soft drinks. *This goes for natural teeth as well as replacement teeth, such as dental implants.*

Food types

One: Liquids. Fruit drinks, soft drinks, sugar, honey added to beverages, creamers, ice cream or frozen yogurt. . Add one point to your total points for each of these you consume on a daily basis.

Two: Solids and sticky foods. Cakes, sweet rolls and breads, donuts, canned fruit, cookies, soft candy, caramel, chewy candy, sugary chewing gum, dry fruit and jelly and jam. For each of these you consume on a daily basis, add two points to your total score.

Three: Slowly-dissolving foods. Sugary mints, hard candy and cough drops and antacid tablets. For each of these you consume on a daily basis, add three points to your total score.

Scoring: If you scored a total of zero to one, you're at low risk for getting new tooth decay. If you scored two to seven total points, you're at moderate risk for increased tooth decay. If you scored eight to nine points, you are at very high risk for new tooth decay. Please contact me at the office if you have questions on how to reduce your risk.

(*Source of original self-assessment is the Tufts School of Dental Medicine.*)

Section 2: Options for Your Care...There are So Many to Choose From!

TWELVE

The "Three R's" - REFRESH, RENEW, and REPLACE.

When you consider brightening your smile, there are three effective strategies. I call these "the 3 Rs." **The first is refresh, the second is renew and the third is replace.** I'll review each of these in detail, but essentially, this gives you the option to tune up what you have, restore what you've lost or replace teeth that are missing or severely damaged. With any of these services, or a combination of several, you could look and feel 5-15 years younger in just a few visits.

Let's discuss the first strategy: REFRESH your smile. This is the simplest, least expensive and easiest way to tune up your smile. It requires the fewest visits and the least amount of treatment. The time, results and cost are on the most conservative end, but it's very popular in my office and instantly effective. Everyone can do it. If you aren't ready for implants, teeth straightening or veneers, this may be the best option for you. Refreshing your smile also includes preventative maintenance and if needed, periodontal (gum) or gingivitis therapy to remove stains and build-up that cause teeth to yellow, fade and increase risk for problems such as tooth decay and gum disease.

Throughout this book, I will share several patient testimonials. I do this not to try to brag or show off my office, even though I think we do have a great team and provide a fantastic experience for our patients. I share these testimonials so you can see how real people, just like you, have seen transformations in their lives through dental implants and cosmetic dentistry.

Former PFL Champion, Sports Radio Host, and Current PAC12 TV Host, Sean O'Connell Shares His Experiences Here at Pinecrest Dental

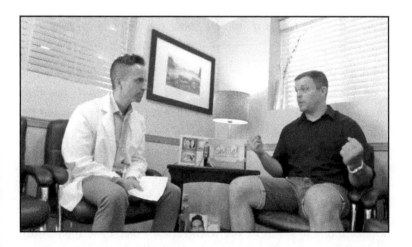

Q: Alright, everyone. I am here today with our favorite guy, Sean. So, Sean, tell us about yourself a little bit.

Sean: My name is Sean O'Connell. I'm from Sandy, Utah. I live in Salt Lake City now, and I'm a professional fighter, or at least I was.

I recently retired as the PFL Light Heavyweight Champion. So, now I gotta figure out what to do with my life.

Q: Yeah, you recently had a big win. So, tell us a little bit about that fight.

Sean: It was the championship of a tournament that took place in 2018. It was at Madison Square Garden in New York City. I fought the number 1. [You] see this scary Brazilian guy, and I TKO'd him. He quit on the stool between rounds three and four. He just couldn't take it anymore. So, I feel pretty good about the win.

Q: Yeah, you crushed it.

Sean: Yeah.

...And I chose the right dentist

Q: Awesome. So tell us a little bit about your experience here with your veneers.

Sean: So yeah, I got veneers. These beautiful white teeth are not what I came in with. I always wanted veneers, but I was real hesitant to go through the process because I thought it would be long, painful and expensive. I came in for a consultation with Dr. Williams. We set out a pretty reasonable plan, and I finally decided to pull the trigger and do it, and it's been awesome. I love them. I love how they look. But, actually, the best thing about it was how patient Pinecrest was with me. Because initially, I went with a more natural shade of white, as you would call it. I didn't like them. After I'd already signed off on them, I was like, "You know, I don't really like these like I thought I would," and I made them do them over again. But he was so patient and so cool about it, and he got me what I wanted.

Q: Awesome. Hey, that's all that matters. They look great.

Sean: Yeah.

Q: So, why would you recommend people come to Pinecrest?

Sean: I know that everyone says their business has a "nice family atmosphere," but at Pinecrest, it's really like that. And it's not just because I've known Dr. Williams forever. The rest of the staff have been so nice to me. Every time I come in, I feel like I'm being greeted by old friends. People take great care of you. They accommodate your schedule. I have a really wild schedule. I've had to change appointments probably 50 times, and nobody complains. They just get me in when they can fit me in. And everyone's just super nice. Going to the dentist is usually an unpleasant experience, but at Pinecrest, it's not. I promise.

Q: Well, thank you. We love having you here as a patient.

Here are six great ways to REFRESH your smile.

The first one is whitening.

You have several options to whiten your teeth. In my office, we offer three different packages for whitening. These include 1). In-office power whitening. This is where you come to the office for an hour or so and we apply several coats of a very powerful whitening agent directly to your teeth after we put a protective coating on your gums and lips. You'll be hanging out in our chair for a while, so bring some headphones, or you can watch a movie on one of our tablets. This option is painless but some people will have some slight sensitivity, so we place a sensitizing agent afterwards, or you can use your home trays or your home sensitizing toothpaste. If you have a special event like a wedding or graduation where you'll be taking photos, this is the quickest way to take the color and shade of your teeth up multiple levels o f brightness in one quick visit.

2). Another option for whitening is a quick boost. This is where we place a special clear coating on your teeth that you brush off about 30 minutes later. This only requires minimal use of your time, and it works very well for those looking to remove stains or yellow spots that are unsightly. **It's important to note that with any type of whitening, your teeth will fade over time.** This is because different foods we eat and things we consume in our diet, such as water versus soft drinks, effect the rate of yellowing or stains on our teeth. Regardless of which option you choose, you'll want to do some touch-up over time. This is different for each person. For example, I only touch-up my teeth for about 30 minutes once a month to maintain the level of whitening I desire. However, some people want it to be as white as possible, which may require more or less time whitening, depending on your personal preference.

3). A third option for teeth whitening is take-home trays. These work very well because they're custom-fit to your mouth and you can whiten on your own time. It's also very cost-effective because all you need to do is add a few drops of gel to each tooth when you whiten. If you're using a professional gel, you can do this almost as often as you want with minimal sensitivity or side effects. You'll just want to ensure the trays fit well and you don't overload them with gel. If your teeth get sensitive after any type of whitening, you can also put some sensitivity fluoride toothpaste in the tray and wear it for about 15 minutes. Plus, this gives an extra boost to your enamel health.

Disposable strips or loose trays typically allow too much saliva to contact the gel, which greatly weakens the effectiveness of your whitening tray or strip.

Food such as dark fruits and vegetables, red sauces and red juices or wines, coffee and soft drinks tend to yellow or fade your teeth the quickest. There are other ways to whiten, such as strips and whitening toothpaste, but I haven't found many of these to be very effective in the long run. The thing to remember is that your saliva quickly inactivates any whitening product you put in your mouth. So, when it's performed in a professional setting or with customized trays, it keeps your saliva off the whitening agent so they can work more effectively. Some of the home products such as whitening toothpaste may help remove surface stains, but they aren't very effective in removing deeper stains or discoloration.

The second option for refreshing your teeth is bonding.

Bonding is when a composite resin that matches the shade of your teeth is chemically bonded to your natural tooth. This is great because it is an additive procedure similar to adding acrylic-filled nails, meaning we're not grinding away or cutting away good tooth surface. Bonding is simple because it can easily be done in one to two visits, and our mouth adjust to it very quickly. You'll have many shades to choose from when you have your teeth bonded, and you can see the results instantly. In my office, this is one of the most popular patient choices because it is quick, cost-effective and painless in most situations.

The third method to refresh your smile is periodontal scaling or gingivitis therapy.

This is where we clean above and below your gums as needed to remove dark buildup and stains that can cause your smile to yellow, and if not addressed, over time, they can cause tooth loss as well. If you haven't had your teeth professionally maintained in a while, you may find a thorough cleaning will instantly boost the appearance of your smile, and it will also make any whitening you do much more effective afterward. As I mentioned earlier, I have my teeth professionally cleaned every three months to maintain the work I've had over years, so my hygienist can point out anything that I need to address sooner than later.

The fourth refresh option is dental sealants.

You probably have deep pits or grooves in your back teeth; most of us do. During development in your mother's womb, and then as children, your teeth form together as lobes. As they fuse during the development process, you get natural folds or grooves in your teeth that pick up staining and bacteria that are difficult to remove on your own. Even most toothbrushes can't get into many of these grooves, especially on back or molar teeth. Sealants are generally placed in adult teeth at age six through adulthood, but they can be placed in baby teeth as well for someone who's at high risk for decay. In fact, I've sealed both baby teeth and adult teeth on my own children to add an extra level of protection in their mouths from all the starches and sticky foods that are found in most diets today.

New studies have shown sealants can provide up to 15 years of protection. Sealants cost a fraction of a filling and thousands less than a root canal. Sealants are also placed painlessly because we lightly polish the grooves in your teeth to remove the stains and bacteria. Then, we use a bonding process to seal the resin to your teeth. Not only does it make them glassy smooth and add extra strength, but it also makes them whiter. The sealant material is a milky white shade that blends in with your teeth while covering up many stains or discolorations.

I had several of my molar teeth sealed as a child, and over the past 10 years, I've had a few of them resealed and updated. The sealing coating is very thin and not noticeable. You probably need your sealants touched up or replaced every three to 20 years depending on how well you maintain them, the food you eat and your home hygiene habits. The sealant coating can only be applied very thinly to avoid interfering with our bite. It can wear over time, but the cost savings are substantial and your quality of life will be much improved. Plus, as a bonus, it brightens the look of your teeth.

A fifth option for refreshing your smile is to replace old silver fillings or metal crowns.

Silver fillings have been very controversial for many years, but the silver itself is not necessarily bad for our teeth. The concern is how the silver is disposed of when it is removed from our teeth. Older crowns have metal underneath or are completely made of gold. Although they can last for many years and the metal is generally not harmful, unless it is made of low-grade metals such as nickel, many people do not like the look or the gray appearance of the gum line. Replacing these with newer ceramics and composites can brighten a smile as well as save and strengthen your teeth. Usually, you'll start to notice a change in color on these teeth when they need to be replaced, or your dentist will find cracks or leaks underneath them, which means they need to be replaced ASAP or you could develop a root infection in no time.

The sixth way to refresh your smile is to have your wisdom teeth removed.

Wisdom teeth removal has also been controversial because many people wonder why we even have them if we don't need them? Many also wonder if they can crowd out their teeth or cause other teeth to shift and get gaps. There are several theories to the reason we have wisdom teeth. One theory is that, as our diets have become more processed, our mouths are not as big and strong as they used to be so we don't have the room for wisdom teeth that we did centuries ago. Another school of thought is that before there were better ways to replace and save our teeth, we may have needed those wisdom teeth in case we had to have other teeth pulled the old-fashioned way, which would greatly hamper your ability to chew. Fortunately those days are gone, but we still remove a lot of wisdom teeth.

Wisdom teeth are simply too much maintenance for most people, even if they were told they have enough room. Many of us struggle with flossing or brushing our wisdom teeth because they are so far back there and harder to clean underneath the gums. If you are one of many adults with a history of gum disease or tooth decay, you'll likely need to floss two or more times per day if you decide to save your wisdom teeth. That's a big reason why many people elect to have them removed; they don't want to deal with extra maintenance. If you've had any issues with your wisdom teeth, then you should have them evaluated. If you know you need them out but they're not causing any problems, that means now is the best time. I've seen too many infections, some of which have become life-threatening or severe for people who have put off or delayed having a wisdom tooth removed. When they don't hurt, that's the best time to have them out because you'll recover quicker.

THIRTEEN

Smile Treatment Strategy Number Two: RENEW Your Teeth to Great Health

Replacing your broken or missing teeth with dental implants is a fantastic option. However, it is not the only fantastic option. I've witnessed firsthand the life-changing effects of dental implants, but I've also witnessed firsthand the life-changing effects of restoring broken, cracked or dark teeth. Several years ago, one of my own teeth developed an abscess from work that had been done years prior. I experienced my first root canal and everything went smooth, but I'll be honest: when the tooth started to hurt, I considered having it removed and replaced with an implant. Why wouldn't I consider that? I was already involved in both restorative and dental implant procedures in my own practice.

However, renewing the tooth was the best option for my situation, and the tooth has lasted for years. I'm very glad that

I decided to save the tooth and thankful for the experience because now I better know how to describe the options to you by experiencing it firsthand. The moral of the story is this: preserve your great teeth, save your good teeth and replace your bad or missing teeth.

Up next, we'll cover the five common treatments we use to RENEW your teeth.

Kelley Shares Her Thoughts about Pinecrest Dental

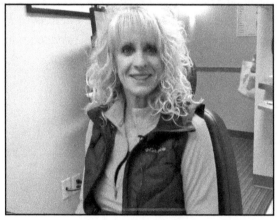

Q: I'm here with..
Kelley: Kelley West.

Q: Hi, Kelley.
Kelley: Hi.

Q: What are some great experiences you've had here at Pinecrest Dental?
Kelley: I love coming to Dr. Williams because he lets me make my own decisions and lets me be in control of my dental plan. He also

makes me feel super comfortable and super relaxed, because I've had some bad experiences. We used to go to a family member who was our dentist, so I was apprehensive to change, but I love that my husband and I made the change. I'm always really nervous that I'll feel pain, but there's never any pain. So, I have had just a positive experience. I love the front office. They make me feel like I'm at home.

Q: Good. We're so glad. Why would you recommend us to other people?

Kelley: Because Dr. Williams is efficient. He's fast. He gets you in the office in a timely manner, and he really puts you at ease. He's got a really good bedside manner, besides his professional abilities.

Q: Good. Thank you for sharing your thoughts.

Kelley: You're welcome.

FOURTEEN

Are Short-Term Cosmetic Braces Right for You?

The first of five common treatments we use to renew your teeth, which is still underutilized but has gained much popularity in the past few years, is orthodontics and straightening of adult teeth. That's right, braces aren't just for kids and teens anymore, and they don't have to look metal anymore. Thanks to new technology, such as Invisalign, short-term braces and clear brackets, we can now move teeth quicker and more efficiently and more comfortably than ever before. Plus, with cosmetic straightening options, you don't have to look like a teenager with metal braces to get your teeth lined up just the way you want them. This is heavily underutilized because in our impatient world, we often want things fixed in one day.

Although it's possible, often it's too aggressive to do everything in one visit. And with options like straightening, it's amazing how we can take teeth that may have a bad appearance or crooked bite or gaps between them and move them into their ideal position.

Not only does this create instant whitening by closing the gaps, but it makes teeth easier to maintain and clean over your lifetime. In fact, this is such a great option, I decided to have it done personally back in 2014. My wife still remarks on how great my teeth look after having cosmetic braces to straighten my teeth.

Quite often, we begin by straightening teeth as the first step, then by bonding chipped or cracked teeth as the second step. Finally, we replace one or more missing teeth with dental implants as the final step. Phasing out treatment like this can often be done in as little as six months or sometimes it takes a year or more depending on your comfort level, budget and expected outcomes. Just like a car that's out of alignment, no matter how great the wheels and tires are that you put on the car, it still won't ride perfectly or last as long if the alignment is off. Your teeth are much the same. In fact, the alignment may be even more important because this one set of teeth you have needs to last a lifetime.

Never think you're too old for braces.

Recently, I completed some braces for a patient of mine right before his 71st birthday. You canhear about his experience on my website, but it's also important to mention that the results exceeded his expectations. He had very nice teeth, they had just become crooked and twisted over the years. He didn't need any dental implants or crowns; he just needed the teeth moved into the proper position and some minor bonding to tweak the final results, and he was done in six months. But he's not the oldest patient we've straightened teeth on. Just remember, you're never too old to be healthier and to have a better quality of life. To learn if teeth straightening is right for you, you can visit my website to learn more. Visit pinecrestdds.com/implant-book-bonuses to learn more.

Linden Shares His Clear Braces Experience

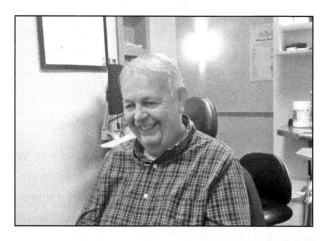

Pinecrest Dental Review with Linden

PD: So, state your name.

L: My name is Linden Mecham.

PD: What do you like about Pinecrest Dental?

L: They treat you as a person, and they take care of your teeth. They make sure you have the most satisfaction, and everything the doctor has done for my teeth has exceeded my expectations. Being seventy years old, I decided to put on new braces, and he actually took care of the whole mouth, top and bottom. If you saw my before and after pictures, you'd understand why Dr. Williams is now my dentist and why you'd want to come see him. He's just awesome.

PD: Super great! Why would you refer your friends and family here?

L: Because he knows his stuff, and he has people skills. He has a staff that is courteous, and they know how to make you feel comfortable. They are consistent, and they care. To sum up, they provide care that never quits.

PD: Tell us about your experience with your braces.

L: There were good experiences, but not until the tail-end. It's an ordeal; it's not a piece of cake. My children had braces, and they got no sympathy from me because I was paying the bill. And now I get no sympathy from them because I'm still paying the bill.

PD: But the results are what you wanted?

L: Oh, they exceeded my expectations. I had confidence Dr. Williams could do what he did, but I still think he went above and beyond. There's a science to straightening teeth. He studied what he knows and the more experience the more he's capable and confident, and he cares and is considerate.

PD: Alright, well thanks for sharing your words with us, Linden.

Take your cosmetic braces self-assessment.

Write down how many of these questions you answer yes to, then score yourself.

1. Are your teeth crowded, or do you have an overbite?

2. Do you have gaps or spaces between any of your teeth?

3. Are you embarrassed about a yellowing smile?

4. Is it difficult to clean between any of your teeth due to poor alignment or crookedness?

5. Have your teeth yellowed or stained more recently?

6. Does build-up (plaque) stick to your teeth frequently, such as on the back of your front teeth, top and/or bottom?

7. Do you have teeth that lean or stick out more than you'd like?

8. Do you have teeth that are pushed back too much?

9. Have you noticed recent shifting or movement of your teeth in the last 1-3 years?

10. Are you willing to wear clear braces or a clear appliance for the next 6-9 months?

Score yourself:

1-3 "yes" answers: You may get the results you want simply by whitening your teeth, having them bonded, and/or receiving a thorough and complete oral health exam and checkup.

4-6 "yes" answers: You are a great candidate for Six-Month Smiles or clear braces!

7-9 "yes" answers: You are a great candidate for Six-Month Smiles or clear braces! In addition, some bonding, veneers, and/or whitening may further enhance your results.

10 "yes" answers: You may be a great candidate for Six-Month Smiles or clear braces; however, further evaluation or implant consultation may be needed first.

I have been a certified Six-Month Smiles and Invisalign provider for years, and by visiting our website (pinecrestdds.com/implant-book-bonuses), you can learn more about the different straightening options we offer.

FIFTEEN

What About "Veneers?"

The second option for renewing your teeth to natural beauty and function includes porcelain veneers, ceramics, crowns and onlays. Today, we have a wide array of different materials, including porcelain ceramic and resin that can bond or be cemented to enhance your smile and restore loss from wear, misalignment or decay. Plus, we now have the ability to make a digital model of your smile beforehand so you can preview the changes and be precision-fit, and the look of these modern restorations are unbelievable.

Many times, to get the best result, we need to restore multiple teeth so things work together in harmony. Imagine you're driving down the road and you've run over a sharp nail, resulting in a flat tire. You put on your spare, which is much smaller, so your car rides a little bit funny. Now imagine going to get that tire replaced and your only option is a tire that's bigger than the other three. How do you think the car would ride and feel? Probably not too great. It's much the same in our mouths when we've had years of wear or erosion of our teeth and we try to just repair one or two spots. It can work but it may not bring about the change you're looking for. In cases like this, we'll take a series of photos of your teeth so we can look at your options together and provide you with a full smile assessment before we begin, just like the architect or engineer who draws up a blueprint before the construction or remodeling of your home or office. The new porcelain materials prevent the gray or dark lines that are common on old crowns, so you'll get years of a confident smile with your new enhancement.

SIXTEEN

Gum Therapy

A third type of effective renewal procedure is gum treatment. This may involve periodontal therapy, gum grafting or gum reshaping, such as with a laser. Many of us have brushed too hard over the years or genetically have receded gums. I've wrote about this in my previous book and described how my friend and colleague Dr. Dan Thunell performed gum grafting in my own mouth on some areas that were receded due to genetic factors as well as years of brushing too hard before I knew better. The great news for you is that by reading this book, you not only know your options, but you have time to prevent these conditions from worsening and may be able to avoid painful or unnecessary surgery in the future. Commonly, when teeth have become worn or shifted, your gums may be too thick in some areas. This is where we can reshape your gums with a laser, which has minimal discomfort and heals very rapidly for most of us.

SEVENTEEN

The "Two-Hour Mini Makeover"

The fourth type of renewal procedure I'll mention is what I call the two-hour mini makeover. This is an advanced bonding technique where we reshape and rebuild multiple teeth in your mouth in just a couple of hours. We only remove cracked, weakened or decayed parts of your teeth and spend most of this visit on adding to and strengthening the teeth that have been worn-down or weakened. We use a special composite resin and a proprietary process to bond to your enamel to add life and years back to your smile that have worn away over time. I've had a lot of fun with this technique because I've seen patients laugh, cry and smile like never before. I can't explain how fulfilling it is for me when a patient sits up, looks in the mirror and immediately says, "Wow." To see some success stories, you can check out our videos online. Visit PinecrestDDS.com/implant-book-bonuses or call (801) 618-1501 to learn more.

With the old silver or metal fillings, your teeth had to be ground down or cut away in order for them to stay on. They needed a big slot in your tooth to hold on to the same place and restore your tooth. But today, we can feather and blend these resins into your natural tooth with special polishers that can make them as thin as paper in some cases. The great news for you is this means the resins can be modified, retouched or even removed if you change your mind later or want to do something else without sacrificing your natural tooth. It's a completely reversible procedure, which means you don't have to feel locked into anything. But as of today, on the hundreds of teeth I've done this to, I've yet to have one person say they want them removed because they don't like how they look or feel. It just doesn't happen. You can expect a makeover procedure like this to last anywhere from two to 25 years depending on how well you maintain them, your home hygiene habits, and how often you see your dental team for regular maintenance in the office.

EIGHTEEN

How Botox Is
Used in Dentistry

The fifth option to renew your smile is facial esthet-ics, including Botox and dermal fillers. Newer Botox treatments can treat and eliminate your TMJ pain, migraines, and aging from your face. Plus, it can make you look 10 years younger instantly.

For many years, Botox has been used safely and effectively in many different healthcare applications. Now we are using it new, proven ways to help patients like you who suffer with facial pain or undesirable wrinkles or facial changes.

Botox is a concentrated solution placed directly into your muscles or wrinkles. These areas of your face are over-con-tracting, which causes tightness. The Botox solution we use allows the muscles to relax for three or more months, and with regular placement, it can retrain your muscles to become smoother and more cooperative, to help you feel and look your best. It's like an instant facelift without surgery. Over time, you may be able to go more months between treatments as the muscles relax.

As a bonus, Botox also gets rid of "crow's feet" around your eyes and the "angry brow" wrinkles above your eyelids. It can also minimize or eliminate unwanted wrinkles around your mouth. Many patients like it because it softens the jawline to give the appearance of instant weight loss throughout the face. I got into facial esthetics because I knew it would add more comprehensive service to my cosmetic dental practice. It allows us to treat our TMJ and headache patients in conjunction with cosmetic dental care.

I took part in one of the first groups of dentists in Utah to become certified in this fantastic treatment option. This great new option of facial esthetics in dentistry helps effectively treat the following commonly unwanted conditions:

- Morning headaches
- TMJ pain
- Migraines
- Cluster headaches
- Swollen face
- Unwanted square jaws
- Teeth grinding
- Sleep clenching
- Bite changes after braces
- Face changes from shifting or missing teeth
- Wrinkles, "heavy brows" and forehead creases
- Aged skin
- Gummy smile

If you have any of these conditions or symptoms, you may call our office to request more information about our facial esthetics packages or the latest Botox options.

NINETEEN

Smile Option Strategy Number Three: REPLACE Your Missing or Bad Teeth

So far, we've discussed refreshing your smile with some simple ways to enhance or brighten what you have already and how to renew your smile and teeth that are damaged, cracked, decayed, worn or broken.

Now, we'll cover the third strategy and section of this book, which discusses replacing your missing teeth or bringing back those that have been lost or missing for years. Maybe you had some teeth missing when you were born or maybe you had teeth removed when you had no other choice or were in a financial hardship and could not save them. Maybe they were back teeth that you did not feel were valuable at the time. Maybe now is the time you feel you're ready to bring your smile back to life or to get the smile of your dreams that you've never experienced until now.

Dental implants actually date back hundreds of years. In fact, Mayan Indian ruins have been found where coral or seashells were used as implants in jaw bones to replace missing teeth by being filed down in the shape of a tooth. When the bodies were found hundreds of years later, the implants were still well integrated into the skeleton's jaw bone. In the 1960s, a Swedish researcher named Dr. Branemark discovered the basis for what we currently use today as dental implants. Dr. Branemark found the titanium that was implanted in the bones of rabbits would integrate after a few weeks and could not be easily removed. It was incredibly strong and Dr. Branemark was amazed at the results.

Since the 1960s, modern dental implants have been changing the lives of patients. The earlier implants decades ago were much more invasive and required much more time for surgery and healing, but they still worked incredibly well and were able to change the lives of the people who were missing lots of bone. When you have teeth or a tooth removed, it is not without consequence. Wisdom teeth are the exception because we generally don't need them and often don't have the space. But when our molars or front teeth are removed, our bone shrinks and our teeth surrounding the removed tooth shifts. This causes issues with alignment, bite, sensitivity of teeth, appearance, root exposure and yellowing. Our gums can get unhappy because when your tooth shifts, you can form pockets that can create gingivitis or gum disease, making it harder for you to clean around them.

In fact, when multiple teeth are removed, such as when someone has all their teeth pulled for dentures, we lose up to 90% of our bone volume, as proven by research. Early on in my practice of restorative dentistry, I studied the works of Dr. Carl Misch, an early implant pioneer who demonstrated the problems with bone loss and how it could be restored with implants or bone grafting. When you do have a tooth removed, you should strongly consider having an implant placed or a bone graft put in the site at the same time to preserve your jaw and avoid duplicate costs later on.

Imagine you have a broken tree in your yard and you take that tree out of the ground. The first thing you know is the tree should be carefully removed so the roots do not bring all the dirt with it. Then imagine you left the hole there where the tree root used to be and you watered it and let it pass through the seasons. What do you think would happen? How would that hole look? You'd likely have a huge defect in your yard. Plus, the ground around that hole would likely cave in. Our mouth does the same thing.

When a tooth is removed, your bone cells understand that the bone is no longer needed or being used. That unused bone is taken elsewhere by your cells to other places in your body where it can be used, such as your elbow, chin or other boney structure. But when an implant is placed or a bone graft, it tells those cells to keep that bone there because we're going to need it again soon. So, instead of taking that tree out of your yard and leaving a hole, imagine planting a new tree or, if you're not ready for an implant, putting new soil in and gently tapping it into the hole so the ground is flush, such as with a bone replacement graft.

TWENTY

You Get Just One Chance

There are many things in life you can replace. Cars can be repaired, money can be replaced and forgotten friendships can be brought back to life. But, your health is one thing you can never get back. I can't tell you how many patients of mine have said, "I wish I would have taken care of my teeth years ago." Or, "Mom and Dad never took me to the dentist as a kid." However, we still have it much better than our parents and grandparents did decades ago.

Before the 1950s, preventative dental care hardly existed. Today, we know all about it. We are taught to brush and floss at an early age. Today, with dental implants, our teeth can be replaced. In fact, with the final results, only you and your experienced implant dentist will know which teeth are fake and which are real. Plus, you will be able to eat and chew all the foods you love, to laugh and to speak with confidence. Don't lose that precious bone.

Between studies and my own clinical experience, we have found patients can lose up to 90% of their jaw bone when they have teeth removed that are not replaced with either bone graft replacement or dental implants . A quick online search will show you some horror stories. (If you aren't a fan of Halloween, don't Google this term.) Bone regeneration is still being pioneered, but until then, saving our natural bone or replacing with a graft is the best option. It's a precious asset, so we need to maintain great oral health.

If you would like to attend our next implant seminar, get the details and signup at pinecrestdds.com/implant-book-bonuses.

TWENTY-ONE

All Are Not Created Equal

Implants are made of a specialized titanium or titanium alloy which is coated, sandblasted, or machined in a certain way so our bone adheres and grows into it. Microscope analysis reveals that the titanium fuses to our bone and our body thinks it's part of us. It's an amazing process. I remember being blown away after the first implant I ever placed. It healed up so quickly and my patient was blown away at how simple it was compared to dental procedures she'd had years ago, such as tooth removal or old-school root canals.

Not all implants are created equal. There are all kinds of shapes and sizes as well as components and varying expenses. Just like the huge row of hardware pieces at your local hardware store, there are thousands and thousands of implant parts available today. This is great for you as a consumer because you have more options than ever. However, it can get overwhelming because sometimes, too many options becomes confusing.

Here are some examples of mini (one-piece) implants versus conventional (two-piece) implants. Both serve a great purpose, depending on your budget, health history and overall expectations.

Mini Implant vs Premium Implant

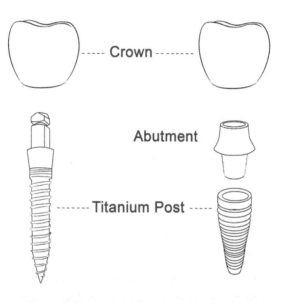

Today, we have short implants for areas where bone has receded as well as narrow implants for areas of your jaw where teeth have been gone for years or teeth are too close together, as well as wide implants that can be placed right in the spot of the root of the tooth that was removed. We can also now expand bone in new, simpler, and more comfortable ways than before. This allows us to mimic nature and not try to reinvent what nature has already proven to work with your anatomy.

TWENTY-TWO

What's the Cost?

Be very careful about going with cheap implants. Dentistry is performed on a microscopic level and fractions of a millimeter can make all the difference in a great outcome versus an ugly one.

I'm not saying you need to choose the most expensive option, because that may not be right for you either. I've seen catastrophes from patients who were sent to my office after experiencing train-wreck implant cases at supposedly "low-cost" clinics or even going out of the country by the recommendation of a friend. One day, a patient was brought into my office; she had been visiting from her native state of Hawaii. A friend had talked her into going out of the country to have her implant procedure done. All of her top teeth were renewed and replaced and she had an implant bridge installed in the overseas clinic.

She came in for her first visit with me, telling me that her bridge was loose and she needed it tightened. If only it were that easy.

Her poor quality implants had caused degeneration of her bone and her nasal sinus was exposed. She immediately started to weep. I felt so terribly bad for her Supposedly, the doctors she had gone to outside the country were U.S.-trained. The thousands and thousands of dollars she had spent on full mouth implants needed to be completely redone from the ground up. This isn't to say that all dentistry outside the U.S. is bad, because there are certain countries who are very advanced in certain dental procedures. However, you should do your research and find someone you really trust before you go all in.

Years ago, my wife had surgery on both of her knees. I couldn't imagine trying to find the cheapest knee surgeon for her. That just wouldn't sit right with me. More importantly, she worked with someone she trusted and who had the experience of doing this many times. Teeth are vital organs in our body, just like many others we need to enjoy our daily lives, so do your homework and work with an implant team you feel very comfortable with.

TWENTY-THREE

Longer Living

We are living longer than ever before. In fact, over the past hundred years, people are living 20 to 40 years longer than they did less than a century ago. This means as adults, we'll have a whole second adulthood. Teeth are very important because not only do they help us feel confident to smile, but they help keep us nourished and give us the ability to eat coarse and healthy foods. You should plan ahead so your older years can be enjoyable as well as the years you are currently experiencing.

Nutrition is a huge issue in our country right now. We consume way too many calories in the form of processed and liquid foods, and this hurts our teeth and our overall health, increasing the likelihood of tooth decay and gum disease dramatically. Plus, being unable to chew can lead to speech problems, pain, and social isolation from embarrassment, and it can contribute to systemic diseases such as heart disease, stroke, Alzheimer's disease, erectile dysfunction and diabetes. For adults, the most cost-effective habits for avoiding unnecessary expenses are regular home care and seeing a dentist for professional maintenance every three to six months.

Nearly 50% of Americans are without dental insurance. But that number goes up for adults who are retired. This is unfortunate because our retired adult population are some of the most in-need people for dental implants. You have options. Today, we have many shapes and sizes of dental implants as well as many materials. Dental implants have been around for centuries in different forms, such as bone or seashell used in ancient America as well as other parts of the world. Today, we have root form implants that mimic the shape of your natural roots as well as many implants that are narrower for areas where spacing or bone is very thin.

Many patients come to my office saying that in the past, they weren't eligible for implants but now, we are able to provide them with options thanks to the many sizes offered now. This also helps because if you're looking for a premium implant system that gives you the best results and the most natural smile, we can offer that. If you're looking for an implant system that is more affordable but still gives you huge benefits over false teeth or empty spaces, we can offer that for you too.

Most implants are made of titanium or titanium alloy, which is coated or specially treated to facilitate growth of bone into the implant. A naturally occurring substance called hydroxyapatite, which is made of calcium and phosphorous, can be found in things such as seashells. Our body really likes this material because it encourages new bone growth. This is why implants from seashells were successful in ancient America. Today's titanium implants can be coated with hydroxyapatite or sandblasted to allow bone to grow inside of it so that it fuses and becomes part of you.

Mini and narrow implants are much the same, and I've used these in instances where people thought they didn't have enough bone or they'd been missing teeth for many years as well as people who have poor-fitting dentures or partial bridges that have broken or decayed. Titanium allergies are fairly uncommon, but I've had a very small number of patients with titanium allergies. If you are allergic to other metals or jewelry, you may have a titanium allergy. The good news is, there is a lot of research being developed to work around this.

For example, a few medical device companies are now making ceramic dental implants that are metal-free. Although these are newer, they follow the same principles of conventional implants and they are a great option for someone who is allergic to titanium. Whichever way you go, you'll be happy with the results.

A recent article from the University of Rutgers discussed the study that was published in a journal of aging research and clinical practice. It found that people with less than 19 teeth were at a higher risk for malnutrition. Clearly, implants have a great impact on our overall health and can help decrease other medical costs.

Another recent study presented at the International Association of Dental Research in Seattle found a previously unknown link between missing teeth and a person's quality of life. The study found that people find it very difficult to come to terms with losing teeth, and it makes them less confident about themselves and more inhibited in their daily lives and activities. This group studied people who gave themselves a self-assessment of their oral health. After receiving implants, the same group had an average self-assess score that rose 50% measuring self-confidence and overall happiness. This is the power of dental implants, and I witness it every day in my own office.

TWENTY-FOUR

Does Implant Treatment Sound Terrifying to You?

We've all had bad experiences in life, and for many people, those experiences happen at the dentist. Recently, I had a patient in my office who stated how she remembered going to the dentist for the first time as a young child, and she came home terrified. Her mother asked her why she was so scared of the dentist, and she told her because she saw blood on the wall at the office. Although you won't see blood on the wall in my office, I can completely relate. I had a scary experience as a child as well. For those of us who have experienced these situations, we never forget.

But today, you don't have to have that kind of fear. You don't have to put off needed care because you're scared of the dentist. Dental care is a very personalized service. Many of my friends have said, "I'm embarrassed to show you my mouth," and so they avoid dental care. Countless patients have told me they feel self-conscious about the appearance of their mouth.

However, one reason I do this every day is because I find a lot of joy in helping my friends and neighbors get healthier, and feel and look younger.

As I work through this fear of dentistry, of needles, or both with my patients, one of the best things that I found to help them is oral sedation. A couple years ago, I offered oral sedation to one of my patients, and after using it the first time, she said, "Why has no one else told me about this in my many years of dental work?" Another patient recently told me that oral sedation, used to treat several of her teeth at once in a single visit, was much easier for her than having one tooth treated at a bad dental experience early in her life where she wasn't offered sedation.

Bryce Shares His Teeth-Straightening Experience

B: Bryce Warner

PD: Hi, Bryce. Where are you from?

B: Salt Lake City.

PD: Awesome! Why did you choose our office for your dental care, Bryce?

B: Because you guys worked on me before and everything's gone great. I've had braces, and I've had all kinds of fillings. I've had lots of work done, and it's always painless, always great. Plus, the staff is wonderful.

PD: Perfect! Tell us a little bit about your experience with implants.

B: It's been great. I don't have a whole lot to say other than it was painless and easy.

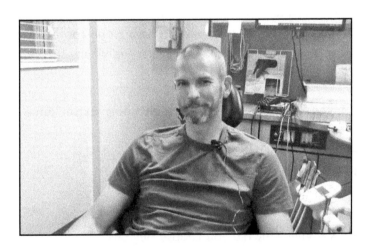

TWENTY-FIVE

Three Levels of Sedation Available to Make Your Visits More Comfortable

The first and very common sedation option we use in modern dentistry is laughing gas or nitrous oxide. It's a very mild sedative. It is safe for most people and the effects of it wear off almost immediately after use. This is very popular in my office because you can drive yourself home after any procedure.

The **second option is oral sedation** where you arrive early to the office and take some pills that are like a heavy muscle relaxer. Even though these do not put you to sleep, you may fall asleep on your own, and they generally make you very care-free. This is the most popular option in my office for patients who are getting wisdom teeth removed, implants placed, or multiple teeth restored in one visit. It is amazing science. It's safe, effective and it's awesome to have my patients smiling while they're getting their mouth worked on. I enjoy seeing those who are the most stressed become incredibly relaxed.

The **third option for sedation is IV sedation,** or to take it a step further, general anesthesia. In these types of sedation, you are induced to a comatose or fully sedated state where you will be asleep. It poses more risks than options one and two, but for the super terrified, it's a great option.

More on sedation will be discussed later in the book (see chapter forty).

With any of these three options, or even without sedation, we will also use numbing. However, the "old days" of scary needles are gone. We now use vibration numbing to make your mouth more comfortable than ever before.

BONUS: If you have more questions on sedation, visit my website at pinecrestdds.com/implant-book-bonuses or call (801) 618-1501 to read more about it or to schedule a sedation consultation and see if it's the right option for you.

TWENTY-SIX

Do Dental Implants Hurt?

Have you had a tooth removed or serious dental work done and you were sore for hours, days or even weeks after? If you haven't, you probably know someone who has, and that can be a deterrent to you for getting dental work done. The great thing about dental implants is because the implant is slightly wider than the small opening made in your mouth, you'll probably have very little or no bleeding afterward. This means you'll heal quicker and more comfortably.

If you've had a tooth removed before, you know what oral surgery is about. In 90% or more of cases, people have said their mouth healed quicker and more comfortably than having a tooth removed. If you've had wisdom teeth out or had to take out a tooth that was broken or damaged, implants will likely be even easier for you.

Robert Brown Shares His Dental Implant Experience

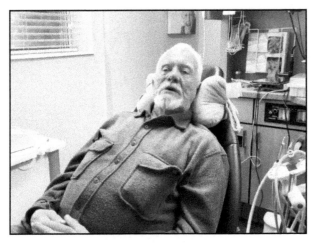

Q: Tell us you name and where you're from.

Robert: My name is Robert Brown, and I'm from Sandy, UT.

Q: Awesome. Why did you choose our office for your dental care?

Robert: I was referred to come here.

Q: You were referred? Ok. By whom?

Robert: My dentist.

Q: OK. Awesome. And tell us about your experience with your implants, Robert.

Robert: It was easy-peasy. It was really nice. No problem whatsoever with them.

Q. Great. Great. They're working well for you?

Robert Brown: Yes.

Q: Awesome.

Robert Brown: I don't even know they're there.

Q: Perfect. And why would you recommend Pinecrest Dental to others?

Brown: Because you gave me a good deal, and you people go the extra mile to make sure that everything is taken care of.

Q: Well, great. We're glad that we can do that for you. So, what made you decide you to get implants in the first place?

Brown: Because it would be easier and less pain and more permanent.

Q: Perfect. And they're as good as you expected?

Brown: Absolutely.

Q: Awesome. Well, thanks so much, Robert.

TWENTY-SEVEN

Another Perspective, From an Implant Company

For over six years, I've been working with MIS, a fantastic company that manufactures and sells dental implants and bone grafting materials to implant dentists. I asked my friends at MIS to share their perspective on some of the advances available today to help great patients like you.

How dental implants improve the lives of patients

By Elad Ginat, MIS Implants Technologies Ltd.

In the late 1970s and early 1980s, they gained popularity through the work of Dr. P. Brånemark of Sweden, who presented his breakthrough work on implant-bone fusion, otherwise known as osseointegration, at the first Dental Implant Consensus Conference in Boston. Implants since have been improving the lives of patients the world over.

Dental implants replace missing roots and can support dental restorations that look and feel just like the patient's own. They offer the ability to eat and drink without the inconveniences of removable dentures, partials or missing teeth. Before the option of dental implants was made available, patients were treated with partial or full removable dentures, which led to bone resorption and ultimately ill-fitting dentures, which don't provide a comfortable or effective solution for the patient.

If the patient needs to replace just one tooth, an implant may be a more effective alternative to traditional bridge work. A standard bridge requires cutting down adjacent teeth to support the new bridge. This means damaging healthy teeth. The supporting teeth become more susceptible to caries, and may eventually be lost too. A dental implant not only preserves bone and gum tissues but also avoids cutting down neighboring teeth, allowing for them to have a longer and healthier lifespan.

When few adjacent teeth are missing or badly damaged, multiple dental implants may be placed to support an implant-supported bridge. This advantageous alternative avoids the hassle involved with the use of partial dentures. It makes the use of metallic clasps unnecessary, resulting in better and more natural-looking esthetics, and it causes no harm to adjacent teeth. The result is a more convenient solution that enhances quality of life while keeping the patient's existing teeth healthy.

Patients with a completely edentulous (toothless) jaw can now avoid the hassle associated with removable dentures. Supported by eight or more implants, a fixed restoration (a bridge) is the ultimate solution for those who wish to improve their chewing ability and enjoy a better quality of life. Implant placement is usually a relatively short procedure, done under local anesthesia. Immediately after implant placement is performed, the bonding of implant to bone begins, and healing takes place. This takes approximately 6-8 weeks. Once this process is complete, fitting for prosthetic restoration may begin. The entire procedure may take as little as 6 months or up to 1 year. In cases where the patient is a suitable candidate for immediate loading of prosthetics, placing an implant and fitting it with a temporary restoration may even be done during the same visit.

New technology

Guided surgery provides the dentist with a custom, pre-planned digital 3D surgical template that guides the doctor during implant placement surgery to the desired angle and depth. Having everything digitally-planned ahead of surgery makes it possible to produce a provisional restoration, which lets the patient leave the doctor's office with a full smile immediately after implant placement. This saves time in the dentist's office and makes the procedure more accurate, safe, and convenient.

Since that first concept of computer-aided design and manufacturing in the 1970s, digital technology has been designed for nearly every step of the dental process. From office management to scanning, 3D modeling and surgical guides, all the way through permanent restorations, the advantages of using these tools are many. For one thing, the productivity and open communications gained by using digital technology to manage patient information is immeasurable. Taking that a step further, it is no longer just contact and basic patient information that may be stored in one convenient archive but the entirety of all digital scanning and imagery done for the same patient, which quickly and conveniently provides the dentist with all the information necessary at every step of the process, especially during those times when crucial restorative or esthetic decisions need to be made on the go.

Having all the information in one location not only makes communication and retrieval simple, but also provides a much higher level of safety and accuracy during surgical procedures, which ultimately, puts the patients at ease. For example, taking CBCT scans of the patient's anatomy prior to surgery, and using a custom surgical guide designed according to this information, ensures a much more predictable, accurate and more minimally invasive surgical procedure.

The complete process with MIS digital dentistry solutions

MIS Implants Technologies has been developing, designing and producing implants, superstructures, tools, kits, and regenerative solutions for over 21 years. With innovation and technological advancement at the core of their mission to "make it simple," it was only natural for them to enter the world of digital implant dentistry close to a decade ago.

Very quickly, MIS understood that the established tools for digital dentistry available at the time were not exactly what they were looking for. In their search for guided surgery solutions, they realized that all other companies using these tools were using key-based systems. This meant that during surgery, each time the dentist wanted to change the diameter of the drill, they needed to change the drill guidance key as well as the drill itself, in order to "narrow" the sleeve and balance the drill in the correct spot.

In designing a "keyless" solution, where the tools provided include all the drills needed for these types of changes and the guidance key is built into the drill itself, the dentist may choose a different drill without having to also change the key that "narrows down" the sleeve. This means cutting surgery time down considerably, leaving less room for error.

This isn't the only feature that distinguishes the MIS guided surgery solution from all others available. The open wire-frame custom surgical template makes it possible to leave the template in the patient's mouth at all times during surgery because irrigation and anesthesia may be administered directly through the template itself.

In addition, the software used to plan the entire procedure, as well as any prosthetic restorations, is highly advanced and unique in its offered features. It's setup and user-interface is very convenient, intuitive and user-friendly and provides a true three-dimensional view of the patient's entire anatomy. Other guided surgery software available have simply taken the two-dimensional radiograph, which has always been used, and digitized it. They don't really show the reality of our three-dimensional jaw and head, which makes for a far less accurate starting point for planning the surgery or designing the restoration.

The comprehensive technological innovations and tools offered by MIS for digitally guided surgery span the entire process of implant dentistry and restoration and offer the dentist a one-stop shop. MIS offers one source for accurate and all-encompassing digital planning, one source for the guided template and surgical tools, and one source for a temporary restoration so the patient can walk into the dental office for implant surgery and leave a few hours later with a full smile.

TWENTY-EIGHT

Help a Vet Smile

It's life-changing to help an extra-special someone smile with the Help a Vet Smile Program.

About two years prior to the writing of this book, we started a program in my office called Help a Vet Smile. This has been an amazing experience and very fun for my entire team. We select a veteran who's most in need, and we provide the special person with a full mouth makeover, including any tooth removal, crowns and restorations, gum therapy and dental implants needed.

A full-mouth rehabilitation like this can be worth thousands or even tens of thousands of dollars, but we happily give it away to a special someone who has given so much to us and our country. The first veteran we gave a new smile to is named Bob. It has been a real privilege to get to know Bob and to serve him.

We give away this service completely free of charge and we cover all the costs, because we know how much of a difference a smile can make in the life of one person. Bob was referred to us by one of our great patients, and he broke down in tears when we told him he would be selected as our next Help a Vet Smile winner.

He'd been missing most of his teeth for many years and couldn't eat well at all with his old denture. I remember he first told me, "All I want to do is eat a salad." This is something that many of us, including me, take for granted, but he hadn't been able to enjoy a salad in so long. That was his goal. When he got his new smile and he talked about the foods he was now enjoying that he had been unable to eat, I knew it was a success.

Our 2017 Vet Smile Winner, Bob:

I simply can't say enough about Tyler Williams and his fantastic staff at Pinecrest Dental. I count myself as an extremely blessed individual. As a 100% disabled veteran, at times I have someone come up and thank me for my service. I was extremely fortunate to have been chosen by Dr. Williams and his staff to be awarded a smile makeover through their veteran charity campaign. For the past several years, I have had very few teeth. The VA had made dentures for me but they were so ill-fitting, I couldn't wear them. When I was selected for this smile makeover by Pinecrest, it opened up a new chapter in my life. Now I have some dentures that fit, and I am able to eat with them. I am in the process of undergoing a smile makeover, which is quite extensive. So far, I've had all my decayed teeth removed, implants placed and more is to come. The end result will be a full set of snap-in permanent dentures and the ability to once again eat real food. Some people tell you how much your service means, but Dr. Williams has actually shown me how much my service means. That means so much. I thank him and his wonderful staff for making it possible to smile with confidence, to not be afraid to eat in public and to once again speak where people can clearly understand what I am saying. While it was okay for George Gabby Hays to have that persona, I'm grateful to be able to have teeth and a huge smile. I really can't say enough about Dr. Williams and his team. I have been to many dentists in the past, but I have never been to a dental office or a medical clinic where the staff was more caring, courteous and happy to see you! You can't go wrong with Pinecrest Dental.

TWENTY-NINE

Snap-In Vs. Screw-In Implants

I'm often asked "which is best" when it comes to dental implant options. When it comes to a removable implant bridge, a snap-in appliance, or a single tooth replacement, you may have the same question.

To replace a tooth or several teeth with dental implants is typically a four- to six-month process. This depends on the health and quality of the bone, where it will be placed in the mouth, and your medical conditions.

If you can have the implant placed at the same time the tooth is removed, or if the tooth has already been missing for some time, it can cut down a few months from your total treatment time. There is also an option to restore or replace all your teeth in one day, but it requires all your teeth to be missing or all your teeth to be removed at the time of the procedure.

This simply isn't right for most of us, because you may have several or many teeth that are still good or that you would like to keep. You can simply replace the teeth around them with dental implants.

If you would like to learn more about your options, attend our next implant seminar. You can find the details and signup at pinecrestdds.com/implant-book-bonuses.

THIRTY

History of Dental Implants

Back in the 1930s, dental implants were discovered in a recovered body that was found in a mine burial archeological site. The jaw of this person was found to have shell and bone carved in the shape of teeth that were pounded into the jaw as an early form of dental implants from centuries ago.

Hundreds of years later, when this head was found, the ancient dental implants were still in great shape in the jaw bone. In my office, a similar but much more comfortable type of dental implant is our most popular option. This is when a new root is placed with the implant and then a few months after the bone has fused and integrated to the implant, we place a ceramic tooth on top of the implant that is secured to it with cement or a very small "fixation" screw; it feels just like a real tooth. When you have an implant like this, you and your implant dentist will be the only ones who know which teeth are real and which are fake.

Another option is called the all-on-4 or all-on-5, which was popularized a few years ago by Nobel Biocare Implants. This is one of the more expensive options, and it entails having multiple implants placed into your jaw in multiple directions and a bridge that screws into the implants; this is typically done in one visit. This bridge can't be removed by you but requires meticulous cleaning and maintenance around it. You should see your dentist twice a year to have it professionally removed and professionally cleaned and then tightened back down to the implants.

This is like an imported vehicle with specialty parts. It's a meticulous but life-changing procedure and has helped many people people receive the smile they've longed for. A service like this chews 90% or better as a full set of natural and healthy teeth. Plus, you can chew on it immediately and smile right away.

You will likely be sore for several days or maybe even a few weeks, but you can do most of your normal activities. A few months after the service, you will need to have a new bridge made as everything in your mouth heals around the implants.

THIRTY-ONE

The "Hybrid"

Hybrid seems to be a buzzword these days, but in dentistry, it has a very specific meaning. When someone is missing all their teeth, the most popular option in my office is what we call the hybrid snap-in bridge. This chews 70%-85% as well as a full set of teeth, but it typically costs thousands less than the all-on-4, all-on-5, or "fix on 6" service. You are able to take the bridge in and out for cleaning, which makes maintenance easier.

Implants cannot get tooth decay because they are not organic. However, you can lose bone and gums around your implants if they're not cleaned and maintained well. The advantage with the hybrid is you can do more cleaning and maintenance on your own by simply snapping the bridge out and cleaning around it with a soft toothbrush. Plus, you can eat things like corn on the cob and even steak, if that's what you enjoy.

Usually, one to two times a year, you'll need to replace some small rubber rings inside of the snap in bridge that only take a few minutes and are very simple to do.

THIRTY-TWO

Who Still Wears Dentures?

Does anybody wear these anymore? Today's dentures are not your grandma's dentures. Today, they look like real teeth.

When a patient of mine decides that implants are not right for them or if they're severely compromised or strapped financially, dentures can be a great option. Upper teeth are generally easy to use with dentures because they can "suction cup" to the roof of your mouth for better stability.

Dentures on lower teeth are usually so-so and take longer to get used to, but they still look great. They just don't chew nearly as well as regular teeth. In fact, we estimate about a 10% to 20% chewing ability compared to a full mouth of natural teeth. Sometimes, we refer to this looser fit as "socks on a rooster." However, this can often be much better than having no chewing ability at all if you're missing all your teeth.

Plus, a well-made cosmetic denture like this can be converted to a hybrid implant system, usually within the first 4 to 18 months. That gives you some forwards compatibility if you decide to upgrade to a more functional option later.

THIRTY-THREE

What's Your Combination?

Many times, we will do combination cases of implants. This may involve a combination of some or all of the following: straightening teeth; replacing missing teeth with implants; bonding of chipped, worn or decayed teeth; restoring cracked teeth; Botox and dermal fillers; gum health therapy and teeth whitening.

Today, with our latest technology, this can be done in fewer visits and more comfortably than ever. Often, my patients will take a sedative when they come into the office so we can get much of this done in fewer visits. You can stay relaxed during your entire treatment.

If you aren't sure which option is right for you, then a consultation with a qualified cosmetic and implant dentist will help you find the answers you are looking for. Plus, these cases can be done over a period of weeks, months or even years, so you don't have to rush into anything. We call this phased treatment. This makes it possible to do it all at once or within a short period of time, but it also gives you the flexibility to take it at a phased, longer-term pace if that is what you are most comfortable with.

Estimates from the CR report find that about 30 million people in the US are missing all their teeth. This number will likely increase as baby boomers live longer and seek to enjoy their retired years. Plus, 90% of patients wearing dentures are unhappy with the fit and are looking for more options.

One recent study had patients rate their life before and after dental implants. On a scale of 1 to 10, comfort was rated at 2.2 and chewing ability was rated 2.3 out of 10. After implants, comfort was measured an average of 9.4 and chewing ability, an average of 9.3. That's a huge and significant increase.

Recently, after placing an implant, my patient Linda stated, "My mouth is feeling great. Thanks for the new tooth. I can't believe how well it fits." This is the reason I do what I do every day because people like you have their lives changed with dental implants.

Section 3:
The Right Option for You

THIRTY-FOUR

What Kind of "Car" Do You Want to Drive?

There are some considerations you should think about when choosing your implant or restorative plan. Earlier, I made an analogy to cars, and it applies here as well. What kind of car do you drive? My first vehicle was a 1988, two-wheel drive Ford Ranger. It was a faded, egg-shell white color with red vinyl seats. It even had a cassette deck but no power windows, power steering or power brakes. It was fun for me at the time because I got to fix it up a little bit and I learned a lot about how cars work.

I sanded the whole vehicle and put new tires on it before going to get it painted at the shop. It was lightweight and rear-wheel drive, so it wasn't great in the snow, but I had some snow chains I would occasionally put on it that made me drive really slow, but really helped me get to school on time on those extra snowy days.

One summer, I was driving to a country club that I worked at as a high school job and some of the wiring under the hood came loose and got stuck around my steering column. As I turned a corner, all of a sudden, it became very difficult to turn the truck and then the vehicle stopped driving and wouldn't start back up.

My dad and I spent many hours matching the wires back up to get it started. Even then, there were some timing issues that we had to have fixed because it wasn't firing correctly. Though I wouldn't trade those memories for anything, I also wouldn't drive that vehicle again, because now I choose to drive something more reliable. That was the right vehicle for me at the time, and it got the job done.

THIRTY-FIVE

What Are Your Personal Values?

When it comes to your oral health and total health, what are your personal values? What is most important to you? Do you value function, health, longevity, appearance, diet, speaking, laughing, and getting up in front of people? All these are important considerations depending on what is most important to you.

You want to think these over when you're having any kind of major dental work done in your mouth. A recent study by the International Association of Dental Research in Seattle found a previously unknown link between missing teeth and a person's quality of life.

In the study, patients found it difficult to come to terms with tooth loss because they were less confident about themselves and felt more stuck in their daily activities. If you're already missing teeth and it doesn't bother your confidence or make you feel like you can't do certain things, then you don't necessarily need to get all your teeth replaced, or at least not all at once.

If you have teeth that are failing, severe gum disease or you have missing teeth and you shy away from some activities, then this should be part of your treatment plan. The next thing you should consider is your budget. A full mouth, complete implant replacement and rehabilitation of your smile can cost $10,000 to $50,000, or more. This is not right for everyone, because it can cost as much as a high-performance luxury vehicle. Although, I'm slightly biased because an implant makeover usually lasts a lot longer than an automobile. However, it isn't right for everybody, and it doesn't necessarily mean it's the right option for you.

If you want the premium package, this is the way to go. Other options can range from the low to high thousands with a variety of options. These are the most popular and common packages done in my office. These can also be phased over time and can be done with payment plans that can be as low as $100 or $200 per month.

We offer some great financing packages that can help you get the care you need as well as membership plans for those who do not have insurance. On that note, dental insurance generally covers very little for dental implants. If you have benefits, you should try to maximize them when possible, but don't expect most of the coverage to come from your insurance.

This is why we've developed some membership plans because they cover all the services we provide in the office, including implants and cosmetic treatment. Another consideration is your health. How healthy are you? Do you have uncontrolled diabetes, high blood pressure? Have you had any radiation or cancer therapy? Do you have any active infections in your body? Have you had chemotherapy for treatment of cancer or bone disease?

Have you ever taken bisphosphonate drugs like Fosamax or Actonel, especially in IV form? Do you smoke or use tobacco, especially a pack or more per day? All these things should be factored in. Although I've treated patients with implants in nearly every category of these health conditions, there are some potential drawbacks or risks you should have evaluated by a qualified implant dentist before you start your treatment plan.

THIRTY-SIX

Is Appearance a Big Deal to You?

If you have a single missing tooth, its replacement may look a little bit whiter or healthier than some of the surrounding teeth when it is restored. For most people, this blends in pretty well and is not noticeable except at very close distances, or when speaking one-on-one.

If appearance is a big issue to you, then you should consider doing some veneers, crowns or bonding at the same time of the implant so everything blends and matches really well. If you're more worried about function or longevity, then you may not need these other cosmetic enhancements, as the implant next to the natural teeth that you already have may look just fine for you.

THIRTY-SEVEN

How Long Will This Treatment Last?

How many years should I expect my implant to last? We'll discuss this more in the next section, but much of this has to do with your care and maintenance at home. Depending on your age, implants may last the rest of your life. Although you may need some of the ceramic teeth and crown components replaced periodically, the root should last many years and even decades if it's well maintained.

I've had patients with implants that were only a few years old referred into my office because they were having minor and/or major problems with them. I've also seen implants that were placed years before my time that are still functioning well today.

It's really fun and rewarding for me to see my patients come back in for preventative care and to see how well their implants are working and feeling for them. You can enjoy the same benefits and have a long lasting smile by getting on a good maintenance program and remembering that nothing is forever, but your implants should last many years, or even the rest of your life, if well maintained.

THIRTY-EIGHT

Does Insurance Cover This?

If you have dental insurance, it's important to know that it is great to help cover with the basics but it rarely, if ever, covers what most adults looking for implants need. Studies show that nearly half of Americans do not have dental insurance. For those who do, almost one-third do not use their dental benefits, which means you may be paying into the program but underutilizing your yearly benefits.

The fact is, 70% of people with dental insurance pay more *into* the program than they get *out* of it. This is why dental insurance is great for basic needs such as preventative care and teeth cleaning, but it usually covers very little major restorative work.

When you are deciding on how your implants will look, you'll have the choice of many shapes, sizes, shades and colors. For example, teeth with a flatter, more square edge give you a more chiseled or masculine look, while teeth with softer and rounder edges that are a little more oval-shaped give you a more feminine look.

You can have your new implants match the natural shade of your teeth or go way whiter and brighter. What most people do is go somewhere in between a few shades lighter than their natural color, but not so light that the teeth look like Chiclets or chalk.

We have technology to offer you a digital preview of your implants and an in-person try-on before they're finished so you can approve the color and shape and decide if you want to make changes before they are finalized. Don't worry. You'll have temporary implants or an appliance in the meantime, so you don't have to be without teeth during any portion of this important and life-changing process.

You can see some examples and stories from successful patients at pinecrestdds.com/implant-book-bonuses. To select the right style for you, I suggest you find some photos or magazine articles of people whose smile you really like and bring those to your visits so we can use them as a guide to profile your new smile.

If you're having one or two teeth replaced, that probably isn't necessary because we'll match them to the natural shape and bite of your existing teeth or improve upon them, but it won't dramatically change the overall appearance of your smile. However, if you're having several or all your teeth replaced, smile design is a key element in giving you a successful outcome.

A couple years back, we had a patient we will call Jenny who came in because she'd gone through many medical hardships and all her teeth had been broken and chipped for many years. She was very polite, but I never saw Jenny smile. That all changed the day she had both her upper and lower teeth restored. She took one look in the mirror and had a huge smile on her face. She couldn't stop smiling.

I saw her a couple weeks later for a follow-up visit and she was still just as happy. She was getting used to the new teeth, which would take some time and was expected because she hadn't had any for years, but she loved the way they looked and her husband was happy beyond measure.

Many patients have asked me over the years why implants cost as much as they do. For starters, it costs hundreds of thousands of dollars to train dentists in dental school. I came out with about $280,000 worth of student loans in 2010 when I graduated from my doctorate program at Virginia Commonwealth University's Dental School. (VCU is a school I highly recommend, by the way.) I was on the lower end of debt for an out-of-state tuition student in my class, meaning I lived fairly conservatively during my four years of doctoral training. On top of tuition, implant materials/equipment, costs hundreds of thousands of dollars.

Upon graduating, I had a great foundation on teeth, dentistry and oral health. However, I had very limited experience with dental implants back then. This means I had to spend many thousands of additional dollars on training and new equipment to be able to offer my patients the latest in technology and comfort to make implants successful and to enhance their smiles. In some ways, the costs of implants have come down because of more available implant systems. As of the writing of this book, you also have more restorative, hybrid and ceramic options than you did in the past, which means you can find a price point that works for you based on your desired level of smile enhancement.

The most important thing to keep in mind is that dental implants cost far less in comparison to similar medical procedures. Just to have the X-rays done and a single tooth removed with a 3-D scan could cost anywhere from $2,000 - $10,000 in a hospital setting. While medical coverage may contribute much more towards your general medical procedures, you are still paying for it in some form.

In my perspective and from experience, dentistry and dental implants are a great value because of how long they last and how much they enhance your life.

THIRTY-NINE

Seven Keys to Choosing the Right Implant Dentist for You

Let's face it: you have many options when choosing a dentist. Maybe even too many options. My team and I at Pinecrest Dental are dedicated to providing a very high level of dental care and patient services to everyone who walks through our doors. I have a passion for elite care dentistry. I offer extensive experience in my team of highly trained dental professionals; we work together to provide our patients with the highest standards of care you will find. That's why I'm sharing this book with you!

Here are some more questions to consider when selecting the right dentist for you: How do I find the right dentist? Who should I ask? What are my best care options? How much will this cost? Do I need dental insurance to help restore my smile?

Here are seven key factors that can change the way you feel about dentistry and help you find the right fit. You should be treated like family. You want to choose a dental team that truly cares and that is accessible and responsive to your needs. You want someone who checks in on you after the procedure to make sure everything is going as planned.

Key number one: the golden rule of smiles. You want a dentist who treats you exactly as they would treat their own family members. You want someone who understands your goals and who can create a customized treatment plan you will be completely satisfied with.

Key number two: a results-driven warranty. You don't just want your teeth cleaned and your missing teeth replaced; you want a smile that will last. You should also receive an upfront cost before you begin treatment. Transparency is key. You should choose someone who always informs before they perform.

Key number three: honesty and transparency using the latest high-end technology. You want digital x-rays, digital photography, oral cancer screenings, minimally invasive dentistry, sleep apnea treatment and many advanced services where you can receive all the care you need under one roof. This doesn't mean you'll never have to see a specialist, but you should be able to see what your dental team sees right in front of you on a digital screen. That's transparency.

Key number four: reputation. Does the dentist have great online reviews as well as helpful videos available for you to view? You should have confidence that your dental team has helped many others just like you with the same condition or needs that you have. Today, some online reviews can seem far from authentic or even doctored up, so to speak. An even better source can be a referral from a friend or a healthcare professional that you trust.

You want to look for someone with additional training and experience in restorative procedures and dental implants. For example, I am a member of AAID (American Academy of Implant Dentistry), the AAFE (American Academy of Facial Esthetics), and the ADA (American Dental Association). These are great organizations dedicated to providing our patients the latest and most comprehensive implant and esthetic services available. I have also been involved with the AGD (Academy of General Dentistry). Organizations such as these usually have members who show a higher-than-average dedication to patients and to their profession.

Key number five: a personalized experience. Whether coming in for routine visits or advanced care, you should always look forward to personalize attention and dedicate a team of professionals at your service. You don't want to be another number or stuck in the waiting room for hours while you wait, missing precious work or family time.

You want an office where your time is valued and appreciated and always worth the visit. You should also be aware of your estimated cost, payment options and service expectations before you begin your care plan. You want to receive customized care to meet your personal needs at a pace you are comfortable with.

Key number six: comprehensive care. You should be cared for by a team who will review your complete medical history, including the oral systemic link, which explains how the health of your mouth can negatively and positively affect your entire body.

Did you know people who have gum disease and cavities are 20 times more likely to suffer from a heart attack or stroke, pre-term childbirth, cancer, and even acid reflux? A thorough medical evaluation discussion, necessary x-ray and records and digital photos will ensure you are given the best oral healthcare service. You should also be aware of your best option based on what's right for you and your long-term health, not necessarily what's best for an insurance company or for the doctor.

Key number seven: convenient location and hours. You want all or most of your procedures done under one roof, right? You're looking for convenient times that meet your busy or demanding schedule, or maybe someone who can accommodate you on your day off.

You also may want someone who can work with your insurance plan or someone who offers an in-house plan if you do not have insurance. You should be able to reach them after-hours and on the rare occasion of an emergency, and be able to schedule appointments or communicate electronically or by phone, whichever you prefer.

You should work with a dental team who understands comprehensive dentistry, not just drill-and-fill. Choose a team who understands general dentistry, orthodontics, dental implants and sleep apnea.

Your dentist should keep up with current techniques and

the latest in technology. Going above and beyond the minimum state requirements for continuing education is a sign of a thorough office who is dedicated and passionate about the care they deliver to you and the people they serve. For more information, visit the bonuses page at pinecrestdds.com/implant-book-bonuses.

FORTY

Have No Fear,
Sedation Is Here!

After everything we've discussed here, are you still scared or terrified of dental implants? Today, dentistry has come a long way and is more comfortable than ever. Today's implants are more comfortable than saving a tooth was just a few years ago. Plus, you have way more options than you did in the past.

Nervousness or anxiety keeps people from receiving needed care. They put it off for weeks, months or even years. If this is you, you have some great options. We use different levels of sedation in my office every single day to deliver excellent care to patients just like you while keeping them safe and comfortable. Plus, the jaw stays more relaxed so you can get back to your daily activities quicker.

There are three common types of sedation we typically offer.

Option one: nitrous oxide (a.k.a. laughing gas)

This gas is very popular because it acts very quickly, has very few side effects and allows you to drive home from your visit, because within five minutes, it is 100% out of your system.

Some people who are not good candidates for laughing gas are typically people who have certain extensive medical conditions, but this is very rare. Most of my patients with multiple medications or medical conditions still do great with laughing gas.

If you're pregnant, you should generally stay away from laughing gas until you deliver your child. A few other conditions include severe emphysema or certain lung problems. However, these conditions are rare, and I can't remember the last time I had a patient who was not eligible for laughing gas when they wanted it other than expecting mothers. If you just need something to take a little bit of the edge off and your anxiety level is between one and four, then laughing gas may be a great option for you.

Option number two: oral sedation

If your anxiety or nervousness level is between five and nine, then oral sedation could be your best bet. With oral sedation, you'll just need a designated driver to get you home afterward because you'll be a bit drowsy or slow for a few hours afterward. You'll also want to plan to take the day off and just watch some movies or nap afterward.

The great thing about oral sedation is you'll probably fall asleep on your own in the dental chair because you'll be so relaxed, but we're not inducing sleep on you, which means it is very safe. Just make sure that you eat a light meal beforehand whether you do oral sedation or laughing gas and follow the prescribed instructions.

Common oral sedatives are Valium and Halcion. Sometimes, I'll add a second or third medication to go with the oral sedation if you're really nervous. Even some of my patients who aren't nervous choose this option because it relaxes your jaw and helps you get numb more easily.

Multiple implants, crowns, veneers, root canals and restorative procedures can be done in the mouth all at once. With oral sedation, you'll just pick up a prescription at the pharmacy before you come to the office. Then we hook a small device up to your finger to keep you monitored throughout the procedure to make sure you stay safe. In all the years I've been doing oral sedation, I've never had a problem, and patients love it.

Sedation option three: IV sedation

If you are scared out of your mind of dental work and you want to be "put out," as the saying goes, IV sedation can be a great option for you. Once the medication is administered, you'll be out in a few minutes, and you'll wake up when everything is done. You'll probably be groggy for longer than you would have with oral sedation and there's some more thorough medical background screening that we need to do before we take this approach.

In my office for this procedure, I bring in a trained nurse dental anesthesiologist to monitor you so that I can focus on the dentistry while someone else is taking care of your vitals and monitoring your body to ensure all systems are working properly. Regardless which three of these you choose, we will still use local anesthesia to numb your mouth and the area we're working on for a more comfortable recovery and a shorter procedure time.

Section 4: Your Long-Term Maintenance Plan

FORTY-ONE

Your Smile Is Restored, Now What?

When you receive dental implants, a one-and-done plan just won't cut it. You'll need a plan, some long-term maintenance and upkeep in order to make your implants last for many years.

Many people are under the wrong impression that by taking your teeth out and getting implants, you will not have to worry about any problems you had in the past, maintenance, or brushing and flossing, but that's completely wrong. If you have an old car that keeps breaking down and you feel like you're dumping a lot of money into it, that doesn't mean when you upgrade to a new one, you are home free from anymore maintenance or expenses.

In fact, some upgrades can cost more, at least initially, because you have to restore or replace years of damage. Your teeth are just the same. When we get implants, we need to plan on how we will maintain them for the long run.

Earlier, I shared a scary story about the patient I had come in from Hawaii in tears because she received implants out of the country and spent tens of thousands of dollars on them only to have her bone around her front top teeth collapse up into her sinus where she would need extensive grafting and have to have the procedure done all over again.

This is so sad. I've had a few other similar patients referred in to me when they've had a bad experience or they've gone to a place where the standard of practice wasn't up to par. Don't let this be you. Do your research ahead of time so you are comfortable with the office you choose.

Today, one in four adults have untreated tooth decay. In Utah, where our population is estimated to be over three million, that's nearly 800,000 Utahns who may be suffering from a disease they don't even know about. That number goes up when you factor in that 50% of adults have some form of gum disease and even 65% or higher in seniors.

These numbers are shocking, but don't let them get you down. Many of us become frustrated because we feel like we brush and try to eat right yet we still have teeth problems. Remember, even a few decades ago, adults had most, if not all of their teeth missing. They didn't have the replacement options we have today. Today, the ADA reports that over 50% of adults over the age of 60 have half or more of their teeth missing.

These statistics mean two important things for you. The first is, work on saving your teeth whenever possible. You should see your implant dentist regularly and most importantly, you should do things at home every day to clean and protect your teeth, including drinking water between meals and having a good home hygiene routine.

The second thing this means is that if you don't maintain this well, then you should know what your replacement options are in the near or long-term future. For example, the situation we run into in my office every single day is one or more teeth that are badly broken, chipped or cracked that will require root canals and potentially gum surgery and multiple crowns to restore.

My guideline is, if it won't last five years or more, then I usually wouldn't recommend it for myself or a family member, which means I wouldn't recommend it for you either. That doesn't mean we don't do it. For some situations, getting just a couple more years out of a tooth is just fine. If that's your goal, then go for it, because doing nothing will only cause spreading disease and decay.

If you are in that situation, you may like to look at other options so you can make a decision you feel the most comfortable with. For most people, replacing a tooth that's in that bad of shape feels much better. You may be tempted to put it off, but then your teeth shift or drift or your bite could collapse, which will cost you even more in the long run. Plan ahead. Even if you do phased treatment, there are ways that work very well and look nice that will save your smile and the alignment of your mouth.

FORTY-TWO

Five Core Principles to Add Extra Years to Your Health

In the previous section, I used the analogy of cars compared to your teeth. Just like your cars have different options, some with more bells and whistles than others, you have options when you have your smile makeover or when you get dental implants. Your situation will be unique to you and should be treated with a customized solution. However, there are some basic principles you should understand and make sure you are prepared for when you get your new implants, or in this case, your new "vehicles."

There are five core principles of maintenance for implants you should be aware of, and I'll go through these one by one to help you understand: home care, professional care, water, supplements, and oral appliances.

Core Principle One: What You Do at Home Matters Most!

The first core principle is home care because it is number one in importance for the long-term health of your mouth and your implants. In most cases, the implants will last decades and possibly even a lifetime, but if not well cleaned and maintained at home, you can lose a bone and gums around your implants or they can become loose and require surgery, therapy, or replacement to get them back to a healthy state.

Home care is your number one secret weapon because the few things you do on a daily basis can do much more than any supplement you can take or professional care you can receive. A while back, I had a patient come into my office who was nearly 90 years old. She was losing her vision and dexterity, but one of the crowns had come off and she couldn't bear to go to church that weekend with her tooth off.

Upon observation, she had a crown that was probably 30 years old or more. It was made of gold, which is less common today, but it was still in very good shape, and she had taken great care of it. She used a water irrigator every single day, and she actually washed some of the cement away that held her crown on. This wasn't a problem at all, because the tooth was very sound and clean underneath—one of the best I've ever seen underneath a crown of that age.

If you do the same with your implants, then when or if they require future maintenance, it will be much easier for you and your implant dentist. Just like exercise, that little bit you do each day will go a long way and compound over the years.

Core Principle Two: Professional Care

Your number two weapon in your five core principles of implant maintenance is professional care. I see hundreds and hundreds of implant teeth every year, and I have quite a few patients who have multiple or complete mouth implants. It's easier to tell those who are maintaining well at home versus those who are not.

When we take out your appliance or look underneath the gums around your implants, we will be able to tell how well you've been cleaning at home. If there's lots of soft or hard buildup, or if your gums are red, puffy or bleeding, we'll know that we need to add some more steps into your home recipe to keep that implant healthy.

Think of your implant like a pole in concrete. As long as the earth around that concrete is sound, it will last a long time, but if the earth becomes soft or damaged, or if it recedes, it doesn't matter how good the concrete is, because it will start to come loose in the earth and the pole will move around.

Today, nearly 50% of adults have some form of gum disease, which includes around implants. Two-thirds of adults over 65 have gum disease, so that number jumps up when you become a senior. Recently, a new study from the *American Journal of Hypertension* found that post-menopausal women who have experienced tooth loss are at an increased risk of developing hypertension (high blood pressure).

Nearly 40,000 post-menopausal women were studied and those who suffered with tooth loss had one-fifth higher risk of developing high blood pressure compared to the women who had their teeth intact. What's interesting is the association was even stronger among younger women.

One of the reasons we find this as an issue is because most people with tooth loss will change their diets to softer and more processed foods because it's tougher to eat coarser, healthier, whole foods if you have missing or painful teeth. The processed foods don't come without a risk. If you're eating processed foods, both your mouth, teeth and blood become more acidic, which is harmful on your body. As your body tries to compensate, it could elevate your blood pressure. This can be added to by what is known as "leaky gut."

Don't let the bed bugs bite. Spreading bacteria will destroy your other teeth or implants as well as cause bad breath and decrease the quality of your overall health. Bacteria from an irritated or infected implant can spread to your teeth, and bacteria from your teeth can spread to your implants both during the day and at night while you sleep.

Your mouth is like a swimming pool for bacteria, both good and bad. If the good ones grow and overpower the bad ones, then your breath gets better and your mouth stays healthier. Using things like prebiotics and probiotics formulated for the mouth can really help.

I'll go into this in more detail in another section, but if you have more of the bad bugs than good, they will swim and spread around your mouth, contaminating and infecting other areas until conditions get worse. One day, you may even wake up with a toothache or an implant ache.

Implants don't have nerves inside of them like teeth, but there are millions of tiny cells all around your mouth; the bone and gums, which hold your implant into your mouth, also contain thousands of nerve endings that feel sensations if the implant is not healthy.

The good news is, you will never have a true toothache on an implant like you would on a tooth, but if not maintained well, you can have issues. If you have implants, you should have your teeth professionally maintained by your dentist and hygienist at least twice a year. For some people, they need to go up to four times a year depending on other associated factors and risks. Your healthy gums support the longevity of your implants and vice versa. They work together in harmony.

Some implants contain many parts and pieces and others just a few. When selecting an implant and your implant dentist, it's important to use high-quality parts and pieces that are easy to order and to work with some of the more researched and better developed implant systems. Saving a few bucks on an implant today could cost you a lot more later if you have an implant come loose or if you need another implant placed and those parts are no longer available.

I've had some cases referred into my office of new patients with implants done many years ago. It can take more time and expense to find the right parts, because some of them are no longer made today. Many types of implant crowns, which is the ceramic portion that looks like a tooth that will connect to your implant, have tiny threaded screws inside them that secure them to the implant. These can loosen over time, which is not a big issue, because they can be tightened fairly simply by a qualified implant dental office.

Of the hundreds and hundreds of implants I see each year, I usually only get three to five of these per year that need to be tightened. It's rare but it can happen. If it does, it's not a big deal, but get into your dentist as soon as possible so you don't develop any pain or strip the threads.

Some studies have shown that cows chew tens of thousands a time each day to mash up and digest their food, which is also why they have multiple stomachs. Although there are no well-published studies on humans, in my research, I estimate that we chew, on average, several hundred to a couple thousand times per day. Add on speaking, swallowing, sleeping and resting your mouth, and your teeth may touch up to 2000 times or more per day. It is still amazing to me that teeth last as long as they do.

When you speak, chew, eat, laugh, sleep or exercise, your teeth can touch in different ways. If you imagine tapping something hundreds or thousands of times per day with a small hammer, you can bet that it would loosen over time. This is the same reason that your fillings can chip, your crowns can come loose or come off or your implant crown could loosen against your implant. Your teeth could touch up to 10 times more if you grind or clench your teeth during the day or unknowingly in your sleep.

As long as you're taking good care of your mouth, these are not big problems, but if you are skipping professional visits and not brushing, flossing or drinking water, you may have some big work that needs to be done from expenses that could be avoided.

Core Principle Three: Water. Water is the best insurance available. As I discussed in section one, water is a key element to a healthy mouth. In fact, the largest portion of your tooth, which is called dentin, is over 20% water. While it is possible for you to drink too much water, it is rare. I do advise that you drink it regularly throughout the day and keep soft drinks, energy drinks and diet sodas to a minimum. My rule of thumb is two or less sodas per week for you to play it safe and not damage or weaken your enamel.

Let's be honest: I love the taste of some sodas and diet drinks, but I keep them to a minimum. I'm what I would call a social or weekend soda drinker, and less and less as time goes on. You may think they taste great too. I used to have 2-3 sodas per weekend, but as of this writing, it has been nearly 2 months since I had a diet drink. The problem with soft drinks is they're full of preservatives and acidic components, which are really damaging on teeth as well as your body.

If you are taking any medications that dry your mouth out, or if you are a mouth breather, or have sleep apnea, this can dehydrate your teeth and make them more susceptible to cracking and chipping. Imagine the dentin inside your teeth like a firm sponge. What would happen if that sponge dried out and then you tapped it over and over again? That's what happens to your teeth if you are experiencing dry mouth. You may not feel it but your teeth slowly become weaker and more brittle and are prone to infection and cracking at their roots.

The same would happen with your dentin or the middle-core of your tooth. If it dries out or gets dehydrated and you chew over and over and over again on that tooth, eventually the tooth can become sensitive, break, chip, crack or require root canal treatment, or worse yet, removal to relieve your symptoms.

Between meals, if you've already had your quota of water for the day, then you should also swish your mouth vigorously with water to wash away the acids quicker. Diet sodas or soft drinks and especially energy drinks and even sports drinks contain so much acid that it can take up to an hour to get it washed off your teeth. If you drink and swish with water, this can accelerate the cleansing much faster.

I have worked with many of my patients who gradually switched their diet to avoid sodas. Their dental bills have decreased dramatically and their teeth have remained brighter and less sensitive. Now, you may be thinking, why does it matter if I drink soda if I have a mouthful of implants? Well, although implants can't get tooth decay, you can develop gum irritation, bleeding gums or bone loss from soft drinks. The acid can stain or discolor your crowns or implant bridges and give you bad breath.

Core Principle Four: Supplements

What else you can do on top of brushing, flossing and using water for a long lasting smile? I prefer non-alcohol rinses with the exception of certain prescriptions. Many mouth rinses contain alcohol that can be used for certain acute conditions or infections, but they should only be used for short periods of time. In general, for maintenance and long-term protection of your teeth and implants, a Xylitol and/or a fluoride mouth rinse have proven to be the safest and most effective in adding years to your smile.

Xylitol is great because it is a plant-derived sugar that has only half the calories of real sugar, but it is not harmful to your body like the artificial sweeteners put in many products that we eat or drink today. Xylitol is a naturally safe antibacterial agent as well. It's not like an antibiotic that destroys and kills bacteria, because that would be harmful if used for long periods of time.

Rather, xylitol turns off bad bacteria; it's kind of like hitting the pause button so they can't attack or damage the health of our mouth. Xylitol is proving to be helpful in boosting minerals in your teeth and freshening your breath as well.

Oral probiotics are another great supplement I have used personally and professionally. These are not the same as the digestive probiotics you would swallow to help with overall health, digestion, skin health, stomach issues and counteracting side effects for medications such as antibiotics. Oral probiotics are usually chewed up or sucked on to populate your mouth with good bacteria to help your gums stay strong or even to overcome gum disease and bad breath. They also help prevent tooth decay by balancing out the bad bacteria and growing more of the good..

Oral probiotics are a fascinating area of development and will likely be an important key to the future of personalized-dental healthcare. If you are interested in oral probiotics, you can call my office and we can send you some more information or a free sample. Or, you may visit pinecrestdds.com/implant-book-bonuses.

Recently, due to overuse of antibiotics, there have been some nasty cases of C. diff developing. C. diff is short for clostridium difficile. This is a condition when the colon becomes inflamed and usually requires medical treatment. It is a nasty condition with terrible diarrhea side effects. Worse yet, some people have to have fecal transplants to overcome it because antibiotics cannot always treat this condition alone.

Any time you take an antibiotic, you should also be taking a probiotic that you swallow to protect your digestive tract. Whenever you have significant dental treatment done, or gum therapy, you should consult with your dental professional about oral probiotics that you can chew and put into your oral environment to help the therapy have maximum success.

Core Principle Five: Mouthguards and Sleep Appliances

You could spend a lot of time or money on your teeth and implants. Why run the risk of shortening their lifespan? Studies show one-third to one-half of adults clench or grind their teeth. On top of that, millions of Americans are undiagnosed with sleep apnea. Whether you clench, grind, have sleep apnea or other sleep-related issues, or a combination, you should consider wearing an appliance at night.

Appliance options include an appliance for clenching your teeth that is usually worn on your upper teeth only, or a dual-arch (upper and lower teeth) appliance to position your jaw during sleep so you breathe better and get the oxygen you have been missing during rest. Many patients wear CPAPs (continuous positive airway pressure devices) during sleep for treating obstructive and/or central sleep apnea. If you wear one of these and you grind your teeth, you may need both an oral appliance and the CPAP.

This is what "insurance" is all about. Protecting your newly restored teeth can add exponential years to your smile. It only takes minutes a day, but the effects will positively compound over time. Sure you'll still need some maintenance and upkeep, but the last thing you want to experience is your brand-new smile to need another major overhaul in a few years.

FORTY-THREE

How Often Should You See Your Dentist?

What is the best frequency timeline to have your checkup? The general answer for years has been going two times per year, which is every six months. That may be sufficient for some people, but with over 50% of adults with gum disease and that number increasing to 65%+ in adults 65 and over, I advise having preventative maintenance done on your teeth every three to four months.

A couple of years ago, I switched to seeing my hygienist in more frequent intervals for my own personal care. Not because I've ever been diagnosed with gum disease, but I've had braces and gum grafting done. Plus, some cavities were restored when I was younger, so it's important to me to have my teeth maintained and to see my hygienist to make sure that everything is functioning properly. If I have any issues, they can be addressed early.

At 39 years old, I know that establishing this pattern early will pay off for years to come in my own personal dental health. I recommend you do the same. Even if you have insurance or you haven't seen your dentist that often, it may cost a bit extra or maybe some out-of-pocket expenses. However, the cost for one or two extra maintenance visits per year are exponentially less than one extra root canal or implant that could have been avoided.

FORTY-FOUR

What the "Healthiest" Patients Do Differently.

I've seen countless patients, just like you, have their smiles restored through dental implants. Although some cases can take months and sometimes years due to time, finances, simultaneous treatment or other conditions, I have yet to have a patient regret having an implant restore their smile.

Many of my patients have multiple implants placed at once and others have them done one at a time as teeth have broken off or have been lost over a period of months or more commonly, years. Even my wife, Megan, had an implant done in her late 20s because of a baby tooth that did not have a permanent adult tooth growing behind it.

During her pregnancy with our second child, she had a flare up on the baby tooth, so we removed it and restored it with an implant. She's even forgotten a couple of times which tooth was the implant because it feels so much like a real tooth, and it's in the back, so it is harder to tell the difference from a real tooth. To see more examples of patient success stories and how your life could be transformed with implants, visit pinecrestdds.com/implant-book-bonuses.

Whether you have a mini implant, a conventional implant, an implant bridge or a snap-in bridge, you have options and you may not even know what you're missing. Plus, there are great financing options available for you to phase out your treatment if needed.

A question you should ask yourself is, how long will this implant or cosmetic treatment last? My general rule of thumb is five years. What I mean by this is, I ask myself if the proposed treatment will last more than five years or less than five years.

If we don't expect the compromised tooth or problem in the mouth to have a good solution that will last at least five years, then it's probably not worth putting the time and money into it. For example, if you have a tooth that is badly broken and will require extensive root canal treatment, gum surgery and a crown, you should strongly consider an implant instead.

Modern root canals and crowns are typically very predictable and long-lasting, but if what's left of your natural tooth is in very poor shape, then an implant is probably a better option. You will likely ask, once you get implants, how long will they last? The answer loosely defined is years. Years can mean only a few years or even less if not well maintained or if your lifestyle or health habits diminish.

Smoking is one of the biggest culprits for implant problems, but other situations such as uncontrolled diabetes, poor eating, poor home care and uncontrolled high blood pressure can also cause implant issues. Your gums and mouth are red for a reason. There's lots of blood in there, so they need lots of oxygen and nutrients to stay healthy. This is also why problems such as oral cancers can spread very quickly, because there's so much blood supply in that area of our body that circulates around each time your heart beats.

The good news is that if your implants are well maintained, they should last for many years, decades or even your lifetime. Likely, some part or component will need to be updated, changed or placed during your lifetime, but the majority of your implant or implant system should be able to provide a great smile while functioning well and giving you the confidence to chew and eat the way you want for many years to come.

When you have an implant or crown done in my office, you receive the Pinecrest Dental Confident Care Warranty, which extends the life of your new implant or restoration for years, depending on which one of our packages you choose. The key to remember is that you play the biggest part in how long your implants will last. The better you upkeep with maintenance and especially home care, the better and longer your implants will last.

FORTY-FIVE

There's No Time Like Now

Get the smile of your dreams started today. Regardless of your situation, the best care possible will never cost less or be more comfortable than it is today. In this book, I've covered a lot of information including my 10-plus years of experience in dental implants. Use this book as a reference throughout your care program. You may think you have this information down, but psychologists have taught us that **we only retain about 50% of what we learn for 48 hours, and then it's gone.**

After a couple weeks, you may forget almost all of what you have learned in this book, unless you reread or refresh yourself on the information. You may not even remember reading this book in a month or two. Like the old saying goes, it can go in one ear and out the other. This means you need tools to take action today. If you are the kind of person who likes to do a lot of research and loves facts, figures and statistics, then reread this book a few times before making your decision.

If you feel ready to go and you're the type of person who doesn't need too much information to make a decision, then get started today and jump right in. Essentially, you have three options.

One, go on your own with this information and do the best with what you have in your mouth right now. Use these tips and techniques to make the best of your current situation and save your teeth while improving your overall health.

Two, make a few small changes with the help of a dental professional and qualified team. You may be just looking to "refresh" your smile without any major changes.

Three, put my team to work for you, which means you can give my office a call or contact us online for a complimentary implant consultation to see if you are a candidate for the world of implant options we have to offer today. We may be able to offer you "renew" or "replace" options, or a combination of both. You may contact us at pinecrestdds.com/implant-book-bonuses or call (801) 618-1501 to learn more or ask a question.

Scientifically, implants work for just about everybody. What I mean is, most people are candidates for implants. However, implant solutions are not just for anybody. For various reasons, some people are not ready to jump in or prepared to have their lives changed with dental implants. Before you decide, you should meet with a qualified implant dentist to see what options are available.

Simply mention this book when you contact my office, and

I will gladly offer you a free implant and a sedation consultation. As a reader of this text, you will be much more prepared and informed than the average person looking into restorative options. We can discuss the three revolutionary technologies discussed here, which are <u>refresh</u>, <u>renew</u> and <u>replace</u>.

You may also visit my website to receive some extra bonus content exclusively for readers of this book at pinecrestdds.com/implant-book-bonuses. I hope you've enjoyed this content as much as I have enjoyed putting it together for great readers like you. I hope it helps you achieve your best smile ever, boosts your confidence and helps you feel healthy and refreshed. Best wishes in your journey of smile transformation.

FORTY-SIX

Resources and Extras

Linda's Experience with Dental Implants (video interview available at **pinecrestdds.com/implant-book-bonuses**)

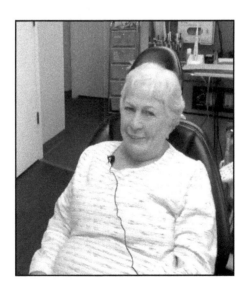

Campbell - Scheduling Coordinator at Pinecrest Dental: Alright. So, I'm here with the lovely ...

Linda: Oh yes.

Campbell: Linda, and she just got a new tooth on. How is that feeling?

Linda: Oh, I can't tell you how nice this is. I just had Dr. Williams, who's great by the way, tell me how they make the teeth so perfect. He put it on and there just hasn't been any problem at all with it. It hasn't been too high, it hasn't been lumpy or bumpy, or rocky or anything. It's great.

Campbell : Good, I'm glad. Have you had a comfortable experience here?

Linda: I sure have. The only thing that was uncomfortable was when the tooth broke off. Of course that was devastating, you know. You don't want those kind of things to happen, but he fixed it up real quick.

Campbell   Absolutely. Well good, I'm glad. What would you recommend to other people about our office?

Linda: The office is great. They were very friendly and accommodating, and it's fun to come here. It's not like the scary old days, how dentists used to be. Where you'd go and it'd take you 10 years to come back because it was so frightening, but this is great.

Campbell: Well, good. Thank you for telling us your stories! Linda: Oh, you're welcome. Thank you.

As I mentioned earlier in the book, I share these testimonials, not to talk about me, but to share with you just how many people, just like you, have experienced the changes brought about by the options modern dentistry has to offer with the help of an experienced dental implant team.

Citations and Links

CHAPTER TWENTY-THREE - Rutgers study
on implants https://www.newswise.com/articles/
tooth-loss-can-indicate-malnutrition,-rutgers-study-says

CHAPTER FORTY-TWO - Health gums and
blood pressure https://www.ajc.com/news/ world/
poor-oral-hygiene-linked-higher-blood-pressure-
studysays/9FWRiEFKbMSE3TCCyUpBOL/

CHAPTER FOURTEEN - https://nationalpost.com/health/a-
gap-free-smile-leads-tobetter-quality-of-life-study-finds

CHAPTER THIRTY-FIVE - ^^ source Kleer.com

""https://www.eurekalert.org/pub_releases/2018-12/ou-
puoww120318.php

CHAPTER EIGHT - Study on Bruxism by Gordon
Christensen: https://doi. org/10.14219/jada.archive.2000.0152

CHAPTER THIRTY-THREE - 3 - phased treatment: CR
Report August 2010, vol 3, issue 8 & Gordon Christensen
2007 lecture in St Paul

CHAPTER TWENTY-SIX - Implant scale: Griffiths TM, Collins CP, Collins PC, oral surgery, Oral Med, Oral Pathology, Oral Radiology Endod 2005

CHAPTER TWENTY-NINE - Attend our next implant seminar! Details and signup at pinecrestdds.com/implant-book-bonuses.

Lightning Source UK Ltd.
Milton Keynes UK
UKHW020807060223
416538UK00015B/1587

9 781977 207289